2nd edition
High-Yield Behavioral Science

2nd edition
High-Yield Behavioral Science

Barbara Fadem, Ph.D.

Professor of Psychiatry
Department of Psychiatry
University of Medicine and Dentistry of New Jersey
New Jersey Medical School
Newark, New Jersey

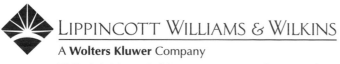

LIPPINCOTT WILLIAMS & WILKINS
A **Wolters Kluwer** Company
Philadelphia · Baltimore · New York · London
Buenos Aires · Hong Kong · Sydney · Tokyo

Editor: Elizabeth A. Nieginski
Editorial Director: Julie P. Scardiglia
Development Editors: Beth Goldner and Emilie Linkins
Managing Editor: Amy G. Dinkel
Marketing Manager: Kelley Ray

Copyright © 2001 Lippincott Williams & Wilkins

351 West Camden Street
Baltimore, Maryland 21201-2436 USA

530 Walnut Street
Philadelphia, Pennsylvania 19106 USA

Printed in the United States of America

ISBN: 0-7817-3084-8

We'd like to hear from you! If you have comments or suggestions regarding this Lippincott Williams & Wilkins title, please contact us at the appropriate customer service number listed below, or send correspondence to **book_comments@lww.com.** If possible, please remember to include your mailing address, phone number, and a reference to the book title and author in your message. To purchase additional copies of this book call our customer service department at **(800) 638-3030** or fax orders to **(301) 824-7390.** International customers should call **(301) 714-2324.**

03
2 3 4 5 6 7 8 9 10

Dedication

I dedicate this book to my husband, Tom Chenal, the hobbyist and farmer who makes it all worthwhile.

Contents

Preface to the Second Edition

High-Yield Behavioral Science, 2nd edition, is designed to provide medical students with a concise, clear presentation of a subject that encompasses developmental psychology, learning theory, psychopathology, sleep, substance abuse, human sexuality, social behavior, physician-patient relationships, health care delivery, medical ethics, epidemiology, and statistics. All of these topics commonly are tested on the USMLE Step 1. Because students are required to answer questions based on clinical descriptions, this edition of the book incorporates the patient snapshot feature. Designated by the icon This feature was first employed in Fadem and Simring's *High-Yield Psychiatry* to provide memorable scenarios and pose specific questions about relevant topics and disorders. Annotated answers to and explanations of the snapshots appear at the end of each chapter.

Because of the limited time available to medical students, the information contained in these 24 chapters is presented in an outline format and includes many quick-access tables. Each chapter, patient snapshot, and table provides a pertinent piece of information to help students master the first major challenge in their medical education, Step 1 of the USMLE.

Acknowledgments

The author would like to give special thanks to Beth Goldner once again for her hard work and positive outlook, Emilie Linkins and Elizabeth Nieginski for their assistance, and the rest of the staff at Lippincott, Williams and Wilkins for their help in preparing this book. The author also thanks Dr. Steven S. Simring, Vice-Chairman for Education, and Dr. Steven J. Schleifer, Chairman, both of the Department of Psychiatry of the New Jersey Medical School, for their continued enthusiasm and support. Finally, and as always, the author thanks her audience of hard-working medical students whom she has had the pleasure and honor of teaching over the years.

1

Child Development

I. INFANCY: BIRTH TO 15 MONTHS

Patient snapshot 1-1. A 9-month-old girl maintains a sitting position without support and has begun to crawl on her hands and knees. When food is put on her high chair tray, she picks up each piece carefully with her thumb and forefinger and puts it into her mouth. When approached by an unfamiliar person, she seems fearful and clings to her mother.

Are this child's motor skills and social behavior consistent with normal development? (see Table 1-1)

A. Attachment

1. **Formation of an intimate attachment** to the mother or primary care giver is the principal psychological task of infancy.

2. **Separation from the mother or primary caregiver between 7 and 12 months of age** results in initial protests, followed by **anaclitic depression,** in which the infant becomes withdrawn and unresponsive.

3. **Children without proper mothering or attachment** exhibit **failure to thrive,** which includes:
   a. Developmental retardation
   b. Poor health and growth
   c. High death rates, despite adequate physical care

4. **Harry Harlow** demonstrated that infant monkeys (particularly males) reared in relative isolation by surrogate artificial mothers do not develop normal mating, maternal, or social behaviors as adults.

B. Physical and social development

1. Physical development
   a. Physical development proceeds in a **cephalocaudal and proximodistal order.** For example, the child can control his head before he can control his feet and can control his forearms before he can control his fingers (Table 1-1).
   b. **Reflexes** that are present at birth disappear during the first year of life. These reflexes include the Moro reflex (extension of limbs when startled), rooting (nipple seeking), palmar grasp (grasping objects placed in the palm), and the Babinski reflex (dorsiflexion of the large toe when the plantar surface of the foot is stroked).

2. **Social development** proceeds from an internal to an external focus (Table 1-1).

Table 1-1
Motor, Social, and Cognitive Characteristics of the Infant

Age (Months)	Motor Characteristics	Social and Cognitive Characteristics
0–2	• Follows objects with the eyes	• Is comforted by hearing a voice or being picked up
2–3	• Lifts head when lying prone and later also lifts shoulders	• Smiles (social smile) and vocalizes (coos) in response to human attention
4–6	• Rolls over • Can hold a sitting position unassisted (6 months) • Uses a no-thumb "raking" grasp	• Recognizes familiar people • Forms attachment to the primary care giver • Repeats single sounds over and over (babbles)
7–11	• Crawls • Pulls himself up to stand • Uses a thumb and forefinger grasp (pincer grasp) • Transfers objects from hand to hand	• Shows discomfort and withdraws from unfamiliar people (stranger anxiety) • Responds to simple instructions • Uses gestures (e.g., waves good-bye)
12–15	• Walks unassisted	• Maintains the mental image of an object without seeing it (object permanence) • Is fearful when separated from primary figure of attachment (separation anxiety) • Says first words

C. Infant morbidity and mortality

　　1. **Premature birth** is defined as less than 34 weeks gestation or birth weight less than 2500 g. Prematurity places the child at risk for **delayed physical and social development,** emotional and behavioral problems, dyslexia, and child abuse (see Chapter 19).

　　　　a. In the United States, prematurity occurs in **6% of births to white women** and **13% of births to African-American women.**

　　　　b. Prematurity is associated with low socioeconomic status, teenage pregnancy, and poor maternal nutrition. Premature birth is also associated with increased infant mortality.

　　2. In the United States, the infant mortality rate averages **7.2 per 1,000 live births;** this rate is high compared with rates in other developed countries.

　　3. Low socioeconomic status, which is related in part to **ethnicity,** is associated with high infant mortality (Table 1-2).

D. Developmental theorists

　　1. **Sigmund Freud** described development in terms of the parts of the body from which the most pleasure is derived at each age during development.

　　2. **Erik Erikson** described development in terms of "critical periods" for the achievement of social goals; if a specific goal is not achieved at a specific age, the individual will never achieve that goal.

　　3. **Jean Piaget** described development in terms of learning capabilities of the child at each age during development.

　　4. **Margaret Mahler** described early development as a sequential process of separation of the child from the mother or primary caregiver.

Table 1-2
Infant Mortality in the United States

Ethnic Group	Infant Deaths per 1000 Live Births
African-American	14.2
Puerto Rican–American and Native American	8.6–8.8
White, Asian-American, and other Hispanic-American	5.1–6.1

    5. **Chess and Thomas** described the endogenous differences among infants in temperament, including activity level, cyclic behavior patterns (e.g., sleeping), approaching or withdrawing from new stimuli, reactivity to stimuli, adaptability, responsiveness, mood, distractibility, and attention span. These differences in temperament remain stable throughout life.

II. THE TODDLER YEARS: 15 MONTHS TO 2½ YEARS

 Patient snapshot 1-2. An 18-month-old boy makes a tower using three blocks, climbs stairs using one foot at a time, and can say *mama, dada, cookie,* and *bye-bye.* When told to copy a circle, he only makes a mark on the paper. His mother relates that he plays well with the babysitter as long as she (the mother) remains in the room. When the mother tries to leave, the child cries and refuses to stay with the babysitter.

Are this child's motor skills and social behavior consistent with normal development? (see Table 1-3)

    A. Attachment

        1. The major task of the second year of life is the **separation of the child from the mother** or primary caregiver.

        2. Because of the close attachment between child and mother at this age, **hospitalized toddlers fear separation** from parents more than they fear bodily harm or pain.

    B. Physical and social development

        1. At approximately 2 years of age, a child is **half of his adult height.**

        2. The **motor, social, and cognitive characteristics** of a toddler are listed in Table 1-3.

III. THE PRESCHOOLER: 3 TO 6 YEARS

 Patient snapshot 1-3. A 4-year-old boy dresses himself with little help, but he cannot yet tie his shoe laces. He enjoys going to nursery school two days per week, and he plays well with his peers. On days when there is no school, he sometimes plays with an imaginary friend.

Are this child's motor skills and behavior consistent with normal development? (see Table 1-4)

    A. Attachment

        1. **Separation.** At about 3 years of age, the child is able to spend a portion of the day with adults other than her parents (e.g., in preschool).

        2. There is no evidence that daily separation from working parents in a good day care setting has long-term negative consequences for children.

Table 1-3
Motor, Social, and Cognitive Characteristics of the Child 1½ to 3 Years of Age

Age (Years)	Motor Characteristics	Social and Cognitive Characteristics
1½	• Stacks 3 blocks • Throws a ball • Scribbles on paper • Climbs stairs one foot at a time	• Moves away from and then toward the mother (rapprochement) • Uses about 10 words • Says own name
2	• Stacks 6 blocks • Kicks a ball • Undresses himself • Uses a spoon or fork	• Plays alongside other children (parallel play) • Uses about 250 words and 2-word sentences • Names body parts and uses pronouns • Favorite word is *No*
3	• Stacks 9 blocks • Rides a tricycle • Copies a circle • Uses scissors • Can partially dress himself • Climbs stairs using alternate feet	• Has sense of self as male or female (core gender identity) • Achieves toilet training • Can comfortably spend part of the day away from mother • Speaks in complete sentences • Identifies some colors

   3. Death. The child **may not completely understand the meaning of death** and may expect a friend, relative, or pet who has died to come back to life.

   B. Physical and social characteristics of the preschooler are listed in Table 1-4.

IV. SCHOOL AGE: 7 TO 11 YEARS

Patient snapshot 1-4. A 9-year-old boy tells his teacher that he wants to be just like his father when he grows up. He does well in school and enjoys collecting baseball cards and postage stamps. He plays goalie on a soccer team and is vigilant about observing the rules. All of his friends are boys and he shows little interest in spending time with girls.

Are this child's motor skills and social behavior consistent with normal development? (see IV A and B)

A. Attachment

   1. Involvement with people other than the parents, including teachers, group leaders, friends (especially same-sex friends), increases.

   2. The child **identifies with the parent of the same sex;** psychosexual issues are dormant.

   3. Because school-age children cope with separation from parents and tolerate hospitalization relatively well, this is the **best age group for elective surgery.**

   4. Children with ill or dying parents or siblings may respond by acting badly at school or at home (i.e., use of the defense mechanism of acting out; see Chapter 4).

B. Physical and social development

   1. The child develops the ability to perform **complex motor tasks** (e.g., playing ball, riding a bike, skipping rope).

   2. Social and cognitive characteristics of the school-age child are listed in Table 1-5.

Table 1-4
Motor, Social, and Cognitive Characteristics of the Child 4 to 6 Years of Age

Age (Years)	Motor Characteristics	Social and Cognitive Characteristics
4	• Creates simple drawing of a person • Buttons garments • Grooms herself (e.g., brushes teeth) • Hops on one foot • Throws a ball • Copies a cross	• Overconcern about illness and injury • Curiosity about sex (e.g., plays "doctor") • Has nightmares and phobias • Has imaginary companions • Plays cooperatively with other children • Has good verbal self-expression
5	• Draws a person in detail • Skips using alternate feet • Copies a square	• Rivalry with the same-sex parent for the affection of the opposite-sex parent (Oedipal conflict)
6	• Ties shoelaces • Rides a bicycle • Copies a triangle • Prints letters	• Begins to develop moral values • Understands the finality of death • Begins to read

Table 1-5
Developmental Theories of the Social and Cognitive Characteristics of School-Age Children

Developmental Theorist	Theory	Social and Cognitive Characteristics
Erikson	Stage of industry versus inferiority	The child is industrious, organized, and accomplished, or he feels that he is incompetent in his interactions with the world
Freud	Development of the superego	The child develops a moral sense of right and wrong and learns to follow rules
Piaget	Stage of concrete operations	The child develops the capacity for logical thought; child can determine that objects have more than one property (e.g., an object can be red and metal)
	Concept of conservation	The child understands that the quantity of a substance remains the same regardless of the size of the container it is in (e.g., the amount of water is the same whether it is in a tall, thin tube or a short, wide bowl)

Answers to Patient Snapshot Questions

1-1. This child's motor skills and behavior are consistent with normal development. At 9 months of age, infants can sit, crawl, and use a pincer (thumb and forefinger) grasp. They are also likely to show "stranger anxiety" when approached by an unfamiliar person.
1-2. This child's motor skills and behavior are consistent with normal development. At 18 months of age, children can stack

three blocks, climb stairs using one foot at a time, and say a few single words. They cannot yet copy shapes. They also show separation anxiety when left by the primary care giver.

1-3. This child's motor skills and behavior are consistent with normal development. At 4 years of age, children can get dressed; they cannot tie their own shoes until about age 6. They can spend time in the company of adults other than the parents and may have imaginary friends.

1-4. This child's motor skills and behavior are consistent with normal development. At 9 years of age, children identify with the parent of the same sex and want to be like him or her. They enjoy having collections of objects, have developed a sense of morality, and are very conscious of following the rules.

2

Adolescence and Adulthood

I. ADOLESCENCE: 11 TO 20 YEARS

Patient snapshot 2-1. A 16-year-old boy, who has a long-standing and good relationship with his family physician, tells the physician that he occasionally smokes cigarettes and drinks beer on weekends with his friends. He also says that he masturbates almost every day. He is doing well in school and is the captain of the school baseball team.

Is this teenager's behavior consistent with normal adolescent development? Should the physician intervene? And if so, how? (see I A, B)

A. Early adolescence (11–14 years)

    1. **Puberty** is marked by:

        a. Onset of menstruation (menarche) in girls, which on average begins at 11–12 years of age

        b. First ejaculation in boys, which on average occurs at 13–14 years of age

        c. Cognitive growth and formation of the personality

        d. Sex drives, which are released through **masturbation** and **physical activity;** daily masturbation is normal.

    2. **Alterations in expected patterns of development** (e.g., acne, obesity, late breast development) may lead to psychological problems.

B. Middle adolescence (14–17 years)

    1. There is a preoccupation with **gender roles, body image,** and **popularity.**

    2. Love for unattainable people ("crushes") and **preference for spending time with friends** rather than family are common.

    3. **Homosexual experiences** may occur. Although parents may become alarmed, these experiences are part of **normal development.**

    4. **Risk-taking behavior** (e.g., smoking, drug use) may occur. The physician should provide education about short-term consequences (e.g., "Smoking will discolor your teeth.") rather than threats of long-term consequences (e.g., "You will develop lung cancer.") to more effectively alter this behavior.

    5. Adolescents resist being different from their peers, which can also lead to noncompliance with medical advice and treatment.

C. Late adolescence (17–20 years)

    1. Development

   a. The **adolescent develops morals,** ethics, self-control, and concerns about humanitarian issues and world problems.

   b. Some adolescents, but not all, develop the ability for abstract reasoning (Piaget's **stage of formal operations).**

2. Questions about one's identity (i.e., an **"identity crisis"**) commonly develops.

   a. If the identity crisis is not handled effectively, the adolescent may suffer from **role confusion** in which he does not know where he belongs in the world.

   b. With role confusion, the adolescent may display behavioral abnormalities with **criminality** or an **interest in cults.**

D. Teenage sexuality and pregnancy

   1. Sexuality

   a. In the United States, **first sexual intercourse** on average occurs at 16 years of age; by 19 years of age, 80% of men and 70% of women have had sexual intercourse. Only about 33% of teenagers regularly use contraceptive measures.

   b. Physicians may counsel minors, provide them with contraceptives, and treat them for sexually transmitted diseases **without parental knowledge or consent** (see also Chapter 22).

   2. Pregnancy

   a. **Teenage pregnancy is a serious social problem** in the United States. American teenagers give birth to approximately 600,000 infants and have approximately 400,000 abortions annually.

   b. **Predisposing factors** to teenage pregnancy include depression, low academic achievement and goals, poor planning for the future, and having divorced parents.

   c. Abortion is legal in the United States, but **parental consent is required in most states.**

   d. **Pregnant teenagers** are at high risk for **obstetric complications,** because they are less likely to get prenatal care and because they are physically immature.

II. EARLY ADULTHOOD: 20 TO 40 YEARS

Patient snapshot 2-2. A 27-year-old married woman develops a sad and tearful mood the day after a normal delivery of a healthy baby girl. She tells the doctor that she feels intermittently sad and tearful for no apparent reason, but she appears well groomed and relates that she enjoys visits from friends and relatives. Five days later, the tearfulness has disappeared and she feels "like her old self again."

What has this woman experienced and is her emotional response within the normal range? (see II B 2 c)

A. Characteristics

   1. The adult's **role in society is defined,** physical development peaks, and the adult develops independence.

   2. At approximately **30 years of age,** there is a **period of reappraisal** of one's life.

B. Starting a new family

   1. Marriage

   a. Marriage or another type of intimate (e.g., close, sexual) relationship occurs (Erikson's **stage of intimacy versus isolation).**

   b. By **30 years of age,** 60% to 70% of Americans are married and have children.

   2. Having children

a. **Normal (vaginal) birth.** Women who are educated about what to expect in childbirth have shorter labors and better initial relationships with their infants.

b. **Cesarean birth**

 (1) The rate of cesarean birth **increased from 5% in the 1960s to 21% in the late 1990s.** This increase was partly caused by physicians' fear of malpractice suits if an infant died or was injured during childbirth.

 (2) The rate of cesarean births is **now decreasing** in response to evidence that women often undergo unnecessary surgical procedures.

c. **Postpartum reactions.** Many women suffer from emotional reactions after childbirth. These reactions include postpartum "blues," or "baby blues" (considered within the normal range of emotions) as well as major depression and psychosis (both considered abnormal) (Table 2-1).

d. **Adoption.** An adoptive parent is one who voluntarily becomes the legal parent of a child who is not his or her genetic offspring. Children should be told that they are adopted as soon as they understand language and at the **earliest age possible.**

III. MIDDLE ADULTHOOD: 40 TO 65 YEARS

Patient snapshot 2-3. A successful 50-year-old engineer tells her internist that she just bought an expensive sports car. In explaining her purchase she says, "I realized that I better get the things I've always wanted now, because I'm not getting any younger."

Is this woman's emotional response commonly seen in people of her age group? (see III B 1)

Table 2-1
Postpartum Maternal Reactions

Reaction	Incidence	Characteristics	Physician Intervention
Postpartum "blues"	33%–50%	• Feelings of sadness and tearfulness • Symptoms last up to 1 week after delivery	• Support • Practical advice about child care
Major depression	5%–10%	• Feelings of hopelessness and helplessness • Lack of pleasure or interest in usual activities • Symptoms usually begin within 4 weeks after delivery	• Antidepressant medication • Frequent scheduled visits
Postpartum psychosis	0.1%–0.2%	• Hallucinations and/or delusions • Mother may harm infant • Symptoms usually begin 2 to 3 weeks after delivery	• Antipsychotic medication • Hospitalization

A. Characteristics

   1. The midlife adult possesses more **power** and **authority** than at other life stages.

   2. The individual either maintains a continued sense of productivity or develops a sense of emptiness (Erikson's stage of **generativity versus stagnation**).

B. Relationships

   1. Many men and some women in their middle forties or early fifties exhibit a **change in a work or marital relationship (a "midlife crisis"),** which may include:
     a. A change in profession or lifestyle
     b. Infidelity, separation, or divorce
     c. Increased use of alcohol or drugs
     d. Depression

   2. The midlife crisis is associated with an **awareness of one's own aging** and **mortality** and severe or unexpected lifestyle changes (e.g., death of a spouse, loss of job, serious illness).

C. The **climacterium** is the **diminution in physiologic function that occurs during midlife.**

   1. In **men,** although hormone levels do not change significantly, a decrease in muscle strength, endurance, and sexual performance occurs.

   2. In **women, menopause** occurs.
     a. The ovaries stop functioning, and menstruation stops at around age 50.
     b. Most women experience menopause with relatively few physical or psychological problems.
     c. Vasomotor instability, or **hot flashes (or flushes),** is a common physical problem seen in women in all cultures and countries. It may continue for years and can be relieved with estrogen replacement therapy.
     d. Use of contraceptive measures should continue for 1 year after the last menstrual period.

Answers to Patient Snapshot Questions

2-1. This teenager's behavior is consistent with that of a normal 16 year old. Teenagers of this age often experiment with smoking and drinking alcohol. Daily masturbation is normal. It is unlikely that this teenager has a problem with substance abuse, because he is doing well in school and in extracurricular activities. Although the parents do not have to be informed about his behavior (see Chapter 22), the physician should see this teenager on a regular basis to follow him and counsel him about risk-taking behavior.

2-2. This woman is experiencing the postpartum "blues," or the "baby blues," a normal reaction following delivery. The baby blues include sad feelings and crying; they last a few days to one week after delivery and usually resolve without medical intervention.

2-3. The emotional response, or "midlife crisis," seen in this patient is commonly seen in people of her age group. She is aware of her own aging and mortality and is seeking to realize her desires while she is still able to do so.

3

Aging, Death, and Bereavement

I. AGING

Patient snapshot 3-1. A 78-year-old woman appears alert and well groomed. She tells her physician that she needs some help with food shopping and house cleaning, but cooks for herself and feels that she functions well living on her own. She notes that although she remembers family member's birthdays, she occasionally forgets the names of people whom she has just met.

Is this woman's level of functioning and behavior consistent with normal aging? (see I C)

A. Demographics

    1. Over **15% of the United States** population will be **older than 65 years of age by the year 2020.**

    2. The **fastest growing age group** in the population are those **older than age 85.**

    3. The **average life expectancy** in the United States is about 76 years.
        a. Life expectancies vary greatly by race and gender (Table 3-1).
        b. Because men are living longer and African-Americans are living longer, the differences in life expectancy between gender and ethnic groups are decreasing.

B. Physical changes

    1. Physical changes associated with aging include:
        a. Impaired vision, hearing, bladder control, and immune responses
        b. Decreased renal, pulmonary and gastrointestinal function; decreased muscle mass and strength
        c. Increased fat deposits
        d. Osteoporosis

    2. Brain changes include decreased cerebral blood flow and brain weight, enlarged ventricles and sulci, and increased presence of senile plaques and neurofibrillary tangles (even in the normally aging brain).

Table 3-1
Life Expectancy in the United States

	African-American	White
Men	66 years of age	74 years of age
Women	74 years of age	80 years of age

C. Psychological changes

1. Although learning speed may decrease and some memory lapses may occur, **intelligence remains approximately the same throughout life.**

2. Memory problems of normal aging do not interfere with social functioning or self-care.

3. The elderly experience Erikson's stage of **ego integrity versus despair.** Either the individual is satisfied and proud of his or her accomplishments or experiences a sense of worthlessness. Most people achieve ego-integrity.

D. Psychopathology in the elderly

1. Depression is the **most common psychiatric disorder** in the elderly.
  a. Factors associated with depression in the elderly include **loss of spouse, family members, and friends; loss of prestige; and decline of health.**
  b. Depression **may mimic (and thus be misdiagnosed as) Alzheimer disease (pseudodementia),** because depression in the elderly is associated with memory loss and cognitive problems.
  c. Depression can be treated successfully with psychotherapy, pharmacotherapy, and electroconvulsive therapy.

2. Sleep patterns change, resulting in loss of sleep, poor sleep quality, or both (see Chapter 7).

3. Anxiety may be associated with insecurity and anxiety-inducing situations, such as physical illness.

4. Alcohol-related disorders are present in 10% to 15% of the elderly population but are often not identified.

5. Psychoactive drugs may produce different effects in the elderly than in younger patients.

E. Longevity has been associated with many factors, including:

1. Family history of longevity

2. Continuation of occupational and physical activity

3. Higher education

4. Social support systems, including marriage

II. DYING, DEATH, AND BEREAVEMENT

 Patient snapshot 3-2. A 78-year-old man whose wife died 6 months ago presents to his physician for an annual physical examination. He is unshaven and his clothes are dirty. He tells his physician that he cries many times during the day when he thinks about his wife and has little interest in food or social activities.

Is this man's emotional response to the loss of his wife within the normal range? Should the physician intervene? And if so, how? (see Table 3-2)

A. Stages of dying. According to **Elizabeth Kubler-Ross,** the process of dying involves **five stages** that usually occur in the following order. However, they also may occur simultaneously or in another order.

1. Denial. The patient refuses to believe that she is dying ("The lab test was wrong").

2. Anger. The patient may become angry at the physician and hospital staff ("You should have made me come in more often").

Table 3-2
Characteristics of Bereavement (Normal Grief) and Depression (Abnormal Grief)

Bereavement	Depression
Minor sleep disturbances	Significant sleep disturbances
Some guilty feelings	Feelings of worthlessness
Illusions (see Chapter 11)	Hallucinations and delusions (see Chapter 11)
Expressions of sadness	Suicidal ideas or attempts
Minor weight loss ($<$ 3 lb)	Significant weight loss ($>$ 8 lb)
Good grooming and hygiene	Poor grooming
Attempts to return to normal routine	Few attempts to return to normal routine
Severe symptoms subside in $<$ 2 months	Severe symptoms continue for $>$ 2 months
Moderate symptoms subside in $<$ 1 year	Moderate symptoms persist for $>$ 1 year
Treatment includes increased contact with the physician, support groups, and counseling; short-acting sedatives for sleep if needed	Treatment includes antidepressants, antipsychotics, or electroconvulsive therapy

3. **Bargaining.** The patient may try to strike a bargain with God or some higher being ("I promise to go to church every day if I can get rid of this disease").

4. **Depression.** The patient becomes preoccupied with death and may become emotionally detached ("I feel so hopeless and helpless").

5. **Acceptance.** The patient is calm and accepts her fate ("I have made my peace and am ready to die").

B. **Bereavement (normal grief) versus depression (abnormal grief).** After the loss of a loved one, loss of a body part, abortion, or miscarriage, there is a normal grief reaction that must be distinguished from depression, which is pathologic (Table 3-2).

Answers to Patient Snapshot Questions

3-1. This 78-year-old woman's level of functioning and behavior are consistent with normal aging. Memory lapses, such as she describes, commonly occur in aging people but do not interfere with social functioning or self-care.

3-2. This 78-year-old man demonstrates an abnormal grief response, or depression. He is showing poor self-care, little interest in food, and no interest in social activities. Even though some sadness is normal six months after the loss of a spouse, this man should be showing some attempts to get back to his former lifestyle. The physician should first assess suicidality. Then, the man should be treated with antidepressants and seen by the physician on an ongoing basis.

4

Psychoanalytic Theory

 Patient snapshot 4-1. A patient has unacknowledged anger toward her physician because he canceled her last appointment. When she sees him, instead of expressing her anger, she compliments him effusively on the decor in his office.

What defense mechanism is this patient using? (see Table 4-1)

I. UNCONSCIOUS MENTAL PROCESSES. Developed by **Sigmund Freud,** psychoanalytic theory is based on the concept that **forces motivating behavior derive from unconscious mental processes.** Psychoanalysis and related therapies are treatment techniques based on this concept. Freud's major theories of the mind follow.

A. Topographic theory of the mind

    1. The **unconscious mind** contains **repressed thoughts and feelings,** which are unavailable to the conscious mind.

        a. **Primary process** is a type of thinking that is associated with **primitive drives, wish fulfillment,** and **pleasure** and does not involve logic and time.

        b. **Dreams** represent gratification of unconscious instinctual impulses and wish fulfillment.

    2. The **preconscious mind** contains memories that, although not readily available, can be accessed by the conscious mind.

    3. The **conscious mind** contains thoughts that a person is currently aware of, but it does not have access to the unconscious mind.

B. **Structural theory of the mind.** The three parts of the mind—the **id, ego,** and **superego**—operate primarily on an unconscious level.

    1. Id

        a. The id represents **instinctive sexual** and **aggressive drives.**

        b. The id is controlled by primary process thinking.

        c. The id is not influenced by external reality.

    2. Ego

        a. The ego **controls the expression of the id** to adapt to the requirements of the external world.

        b. The ego sustains satisfying interpersonal relationships.

        c. Through **reality testing** (i.e., constantly evaluating what is valid and then adapting that to reality), the ego maintains a sense of reality about the body and the external world.

   3. The **superego,** which also controls id impulses, **represents moral values** and **conscience.**

II. PSYCHOANALYSIS AND RELATED THERAPIES

   A. Overview

   1. Psychoanalysis and related therapies (e.g., brief dynamic psychotherapy) are **treatment techniques based on Freud's theories** of the unconscious mind and defense mechanisms.

   2. The main strategy of these therapies is to **uncover and then integrate repressed memories** into the individual's personality.

   3. Psychoanalysis is most appropriate for those who are younger than 40 years of age, intelligent, not psychotic, have good relationships with others, have stable life situations, and have the time and money for this treatment. A typical regimen of psychoanalysis involves 1-hr sessions conducted 4 to 5 times a week for 3 to 4 years.

   B. Techniques. These therapies include **free association** (in which the patient says whatever comes to mind), **dream interpretation,** and **analysis of transference reactions.**

   1. **Transference reactions** occur when the patient's unconscious feelings from the past about his parents (or other important persons) are experienced in the present relationship with the therapist. In psychoanalysis, these reactions are identified and analyzed.

   2. **Countertransference** reactions occur when the therapist unconsciously reexperiences feelings about her parents (or other important persons) with the patient. These reactions must be identified because they can alter the therapist's judgment.

III. DEFENSE MECHANISMS

   A. **Definition.** Defense mechanisms are **unconscious mental techniques** used by the ego to keep conflicts out of consciousness, thus decreasing anxiety and maintaining the individual's sense of safety, equilibrium, and self-esteem.

   B. Classification (Table 4-1)

   1. **Immature defense mechanisms** (e.g., acting out, regression, splitting) are manifestations of childlike or disturbed behavior.

   2. **Mature defense mechanisms** (e.g., altruism, humor, sublimation, and suppression) are manifestations that are adaptive to a normal, healthy adult life.

Answer to Patient Snapshot Question

4-1. This patient is using the defense mechanism of reaction formation. Because she respects her physician, she does not accept (nor is she consciously aware of) her anger toward him. Instead, she is even more friendly and complimentary when she sees him than might be expected.

Table 4-1
Defense Mechanisms

Defense Mechanism	Explanation	Patient Snapshots
Acting out	Avoiding personally unacceptable feelings by behaving in an attention-getting, often socially inappropriate, manner	A teenager with a terminally ill younger sibling begins to do poorly at school and to argue with her parents at home
Altruism	Unselfishly assisting others to avoid negative personal feelings	A woman with a poor self-image works in a soup kitchen on her day off from her regular job
Denial	Not believing personally intolerable facts about reality	A man who has just had a myocardial infarction does push ups on the floor of the intensive care unit
Displacement	Transfer of emotions from a personally unacceptable situation to one that is personally tolerable	A man who is angry at his boss shouts at his wife
Dissociation	Mentally separating out a part of one's personality	A woman who was sexually abused as a child has two distinct personalities in adulthood
Humor	Expression of feeling without causing discomfort	A man who has had a leg amputated makes jokes about one-legged people
Identification	Unconsciously patterning one's behavior after that of someone who is more powerful	A man who was physically abused as a child abuses his own children
Intellectualization	Using the mind's higher functions to avoid experiencing uncomfortable emotions	A physician who has received a diagnosis of pancreatic cancer excessively discusses the statistics of the illness with his colleagues and family
Projection	Attributing one's own personally unacceptable feelings to others	A man who has sexual feelings for his brother's wife begins to believe that his own wife is cheating on him
Rationalization	Seemingly reasonable explanations are given for unacceptable or irrational feelings	A student who fails a final exam says it was not an important course anyway
Reaction formation	Unacceptable feelings are denied and opposite attitudes and behavior adopted; unconscious hypocrisy	A man who unconsciously is resentful of the responsibilities of child care buys his children expensive gifts
Regression	Childlike patterns of behavior appear under stress	A hospitalized 48-year-old patient insists that he will only eat french fries and ice cream
Splitting	Believing people or events are either all bad or all good because of intolerance of ambiguity	A woman who believed her physician was godlike begins to think he is a terrible person after he is late for an appointment with her
Sublimation	An unconscious, unacceptable impulse is rerouted in a socially acceptable way	A man who is angry at his boss plays a hard game of racquetball
Suppression	Unwanted feelings are consciously put aside but not repressed	A breast cancer patient decides that she will worry about her illness for only 10 minutes per day

5

Learning Theory and Behavioral Medicine

I. OVERVIEW

A. Learning is the **acquisition of behavior patterns.**

B. Methods of learning include **classical conditioning** and **operant conditioning.** These two types of conditioning form the basis of a number of **behavioral treatment techniques.**

II. CLASSICAL CONDITIONING

Patient snapshot 5-1. A 2-year-old child is brought to the physician's office for a measles immunization. He cries when he receives the injection from the nurse. The following month the child cries when he sees the same nurse in the physician's office, even though he does not receive an injection. After five subsequent visits with no injections, the child no longer cries when he sees the nurse.

What aspects of learning are responsible for this child's behavior? (see II A–C)

A. **Principles.** In classical conditioning, a **natural,** or **reflexive, response** (e.g., crying) is elicited by a **learned stimulus** (e.g., the sight of the nurse).

B. Elements

    1. An **unconditioned stimulus** is a stimulus that automatically produces a response (e.g., the injection).

    2. An **unconditioned response** is a natural, reflexive behavior that does not have to be learned (e.g., crying in response to the injection).

    3. A **conditioned stimulus** is a stimulus that produces a response following learning (e.g., the sight of the nurse the following month).

    4. A **conditioned response** is a behavior that is learned by an association made between a conditioned stimulus and an unconditioned stimulus (e.g., crying when seeing the nurse the following month).

C. Response acquisition and extinction

    1. In **acquisition,** the conditioned response (e.g., crying in response to the sight of the nurse) is learned.

    2. In **extinction,** the conditioned response decreases if the conditioned stimulus (e.g., the sight of the nurse) is not followed by the unconditioned stimulus (e.g., the injection).

    3. In **stimulus generalization,** a new stimulus (e.g., the sight of anyone in white clothing) that resembles the conditioned stimulus (e.g., the sight of the nurse) results in the conditioned response (e.g., crying).

D. Related concepts

    1. Aversive conditioning. An unwanted behavior (e.g., drinking alcohol) is paired with a painful or aversive stimulus (e.g., medication that causes nausea). Ideally, this pairing creates an association between the unwanted behavior and the aversive stimulus and alcohol drinking ceases.

    2. Learned helplessness

        a. Through classical conditioning, an animal learns that it cannot escape a painful stimulus. The animal then becomes hopeless and apathetic when faced with any new aversive stimulus.

        b. This has been used as a model system for the development of depression in humans.

    3. Imprinting is the tendency of organisms to follow the first thing (e.g., the mother) they see after birth or hatching.

III. OPERANT CONDITIONING

Patient snapshot 5-2. A mother wants her 10-year-old daughter to get better grades in school.

How can the mother achieve this goal using the elements of operant conditioning—i.e., positive reinforcement, negative reinforcement, punishment, or extinction? (see Table 5-1)

Table 5-1
Elements of Operant Conditioning

Element	Effect on Behavior	Example	Comment
Positive reinforcement	Behavior is increased by reward	Child increases her studying behavior to get money by earning good grades in school	Reward or reinforcement (money) increases the desired behavior (studying); a reward can be attention as well as a tangible reward
Negative reinforcement	Behavior is increased by avoidance or escape	Child increases her studying behavior to avoid losing television privileges	Active avoidance of an aversive stimulus (losing television privileges) increases desired behavior (studying)
Punishment	Behavior is decreased by suppression	Child decreases her "fooling around" behavior (when she should be studying) after her mother scolds her	Delivery of an unpleasant stimulus (scolding) decreases unwanted behavior (fooling around)
Extinction	Behavior is eliminated by nonreinforcement	Child stops her "fooling around" behavior when the behavior is ignored by her mother	Although there may be an initial increase in "fooling around" behavior before it disappears, extinction is more effective than punishment for long-term reduction in unwanted behavior

A. Principles

    1. **Behavior is determined by its consequences** for the individual. The consequence, or **reinforcement,** occurs immediately following a behavior.

    2. In operant conditioning, a **behavior that is not part of the individual's natural repertoire can be learned** through **reward** or **punishment.**

B. Elements (Table 5-1)

    1. The likelihood that a behavior will occur is increased by **reinforcement** and decreased by **punishment.**

        a. **Types of reinforcement**

            (1) **Positive reinforcement** (reward) is the introduction of a positive (i.e., pleasant) stimulus that increases the rate of behavior.

            (2) **Negative reinforcement** (escape) is the removal of an aversive (i.e., unpleasant) stimulus that increases the rate of behavior.

        b. **Punishment** is the introduction of an aversive stimulus **aimed at reducing the rate of an unwanted behavior.**

    2. **Extinction** in operant conditioning is the gradual disappearance of a learned behavior when reinforcement is reduced.

    3. The **pattern,** or **schedule, of reinforcement** affects how quickly a behavior is learned and how quickly a behavior disappears when it is not rewarded (extinction) [Table 5-2].

C. Related concepts

    1. **Shaping** involves rewarding closer and closer approximations of the wanted behavior until the correct behavior is achieved. For example, a child who is told to pick up her toys is rewarded initially for picking up only one toy, and eventually learns to pick up all of them.

Table 5-2
Schedules of Reinforcement

Schedule	Reinforcement Presented	Example	Comments
Continuous	After every response	Receiving candy from a vending machine	Least resistant to extinction; response is quickly learned but disappears rapidly without reinforcement
Fixed ratio	After a designated number of responses	Getting paid for sewing 10 shirts	Fast response rate (e.g., lots of shirts are sewn quickly)
Fixed interval	After a designated amount of time	Studying for regularly scheduled, weekly quizzes	Response rate increases toward the end of the interval (scalloped curve)
Variable ratio	After a random and unpredictable number of responses	Getting a payoff on a slot machine	Highly resistant to extinction; response persists with little or no reinforcement
Variable interval	After a random and unpredictable amount of time	Catching fish in a lake	Highly resistant to extinction; response persists with little or no reinforcement

   2. Modeling is a type of observational learning. For example, a medical student learns to behave in a manner similar to that of a resident whom she admires.

IV. APPLICATION OF BEHAVIORAL TECHNIQUES TO MEDICINE

Patient snapshot 5-3. A 40-year-old man who is afraid of flying is put into a relaxed state and then is shown a photograph of an airplane. The next day while relaxed, he is shown a scale model of an airplane. One week later, he can sit calmly in the cabin of an airplane and two weeks later he takes an airplane ride without fear.

What behavioral technique has been used here to treat this man's fear of flying? (see IV A)

A. Systematic desensitization

   1. Principles. Systematic desensitization is a behavior technique based on classical conditioning. It is used to **eliminate phobias** (irrational fears).

   2. Method
      a. An individual is exposed to the frightening stimulus in increasing doses in conjunction with relaxation procedures.
      b. Because relaxation is incompatible with fear, the relaxed patient is less likely to be anxious when the frightening stimulus is presented.

B. Token economy

   1. A **desired behavior is "paid for"** with a token reward (i.e., a positive reinforcer).

   2. Used in **mental hospitals** and in working with the **mentally retarded,** tokens are later exchanged for desired objects (e.g., candy, movies).

C. Cognitive therapy

   1. Definition. Cognitive therapy is a method of short-term psychotherapy (up to 25 weeks) that uses behavioral techniques and deals specifically with depression and anxiety.

   2. Method. A patient's distorted, negative way of thinking is reorganized and substituted with self-enhancing thoughts.

D. Biofeedback

   1. Principles. Biofeedback involves learning to gain control over measurable physiologic parameters; it is based on the principles of operant conditioning and requires a high degree of **motivation** and **practice.**

   2. Therapeutic uses. Biofeedback is used to treat hypertension, peptic ulcer disease, asthma, migraine and tension headaches, Raynaud disease, fecal incontinence, and temporomandibular joint pain.

Answers to Patient Snapshot Questions

5-1. This child cries even when he does not get an injection, because he has learned through classical conditioning to associate the nurse (the conditioned stimulus) with the injection needle and pain (the unconditioned stimulus). However, after 5 weeks of seeing the nurse and not receiving a painful injection, extinction has occurred and the conditioned response (i.e., crying when he sees the nurse) has disappeared.
5-2. This snapshot is explained in the text of Table 5-1.
5-3. The behavioral technique used to treat this man's fear of flying is systematic desensitization. He is exposed to flying while relaxed. Because relaxation is incompatible with fear, he then is less anxious when exposed to airplanes and flying.

6

Psychoactive Substance Abuse

I. OVERVIEW OF SUBSTANCE ABUSE

Patient snapshot 6-1. A 23-year-old man is brought to the emergency room by the police after causing a disturbance in a shopping mall. The patient tells the physician that he is "on top of the world" and is communicating mentally with the President of the United States. One hour later, the patient is very quiet and shows little response to the physician's presence.

If this patient's behavior is due to substance abuse, which substance is most likely involved? (see Table 6-2)

A. Demographics. Caffeine, nicotine, alcohol, marijuana, cocaine and, to a lesser extent, heroin are the most commonly used substances in the United States (Table 6-1). Barbiturates and hallucinogens are also commonly used.

B. Psychoactive substance use disorder is a pattern of abnormal substance use leading to:

  1. **Impairment** of social, physical, or occupational functioning

  2. **Tolerance, dependence,** or both
   a. **Tolerance** is the need for increased amounts of a substance to gain the desired effect; **cross-tolerance** occurs when tolerance develops to one substance as the result of use of another substance.
   b. **Dependence** is the abuse of a substance plus tolerance, withdrawal symptoms, or a pattern of repetitive use. The effects of use and withdrawal of substances are listed in Table 6-2.

II. NEUROTRANSMITTER ASSOCIATIONS

A. Stimulants work primarily by increasing the availability of **dopamine and glutamate.**

  1. Amphetamine use causes the release of dopamine. Cocaine blocks the reuptake of dopamine.

  2. Increased availability of dopamine in the synapse is apparently involved in the **"reward system"** of the brain and the euphoric effects of stimulants and opiates. As in schizophrenia (see Chapter 11), increased dopamine availability may also result in **psychotic symptoms.**

B. Sedative agents work primarily by increasing the activity of the inhibitory neurotransmitter γ-aminobutyric acid **(GABA).**

Table 6-1
Demographics and Characteristics of Commonly Used Substances in the United States

Substance (Lifetime Prevalence, Nonclinical Use)	Comments
Alcohol (85%)	• 10%–13% lifetime prevalence of abuse or dependence • Increased use among Native Americans and Eskimos • 2:1 male-to-female ratio of abuse • Associated with automobile accidents, homicide, suicide, rape, child physical and sexual abuse, spousal and elder abuse, childhood ADHD and conduct disorder, liver dysfunction, gastrointestinal problems (e.g., ulcers), hallucinations, thiamine deficiency, as well as Korsakoff, Wernicke, and fetal alcohol syndromes
Caffeine (80%)	• Found in coffee (125 mg/cup), tea (65 mg/cup), cola (40 mg/cup), nonprescription stimulants, and over-the counter diet agents
Nicotine (55%)	• Increased smoking among teenagers, African-Americans, and women • Associated with cancer of the lung, pharynx, and bladder • Associated with cardiovascular diseases • Decreases life expectancy more than any other substance
Marijuana (33%)	• Most commonly used illegal psychoactive substance • Current increased use in 12 to 25 year olds • Primary active compound is tetrahydrocannabinol (THC)
Cocaine (12%)	• "Crack" and "freebase" are cheap, smokable forms • In pure form, it is sniffed into the nose ("snorted") • Cocaine use peaked in 1985 and has since declined • Hyperactivity and growth retardation are seen in newborns of users
Amphetamines (7%)	• Used clinically in the treatment of ADHD, narcolepsy (see Chapter 7), depression, and obesity; clinical formulations include dextroamphetamine (Dexedrine), methamphetamine (Desoxyn), and methylphenidate (Ritalin) • "Speed," "ice" (methamphetamine), and "ecstasy" (MDMA) are street names for amphetamine compounds.
Heroin (7%)	• Is more potent, crosses the blood-brain barrier faster, has a faster onset of action, and more euphoric effect than medically used opiates (e.g., morphine) • Higher rate of use in large cities; use is increasing • Intravenous use is associated with transmission of HIV
Benzodiazepines and barbiturates (4%)	• Used clinically as antianxiety agents, sedatives, muscle relaxants, anticonvulsants, and anesthetics; long-acting agents are used to treat alcohol withdrawal
Hallucinogens (3%)	• LSD is ingested • PCP is typically smoked in a marijuana or other cigarette

ADHD = attention deficit hyperactivity disorder; LSD = lysergic acid diethylamide; MDMA = methylene dioxymethamphetamine; PCP = phencyclidine.

Table 6-2
Effects of Use and Withdrawal of Psychoactive Substances

Category	Effects of Use	Effects of Withdrawal
Sedatives • Alcohol • Benzodiazepines • Barbiturates	• Mood elevation, decreased anxiety, sedation, behavioral disinhibition, respiratory depression • Barbiturates have a low safety margin; benzodiazepines have a high safety margin.	• Mood depression, increased anxiety, tremor, insomnia, seizures, cardiovascular collapse, and psychotic symptoms such as formication (i.e., tactile hallucinations of bugs crawling on the skin) • Is called delirium tremens (the "DTs") when associated with alcohol withdrawal • Hospitalization is necessary for withdrawal in all heavy or long-term users.
Opioids • Heroin • Methadone • Opioids used medically (e.g., morphine)	• Mood elevation, sedation, analgesia, respiratory depression, constipation, pupil constriction	• Mood depression, anxiety, sweating, fever, rhinorrhea, piloerection, yawning, diarrhea, pupil dilation • Death from withdrawal is rare.
Stimulants **Major stimulants** • Amphetamines • Cocaine **Minor stimulants** • Caffeine • Nicotine	• Mood elevation, insomnia, increased cardiovascular, neurological, and gastrointestinal activity, pupil dilation • Psychotic symptoms, including formication (e.g., "cocaine bugs"), with use of major stimulants	• Mood depression, lethargy, increased appetite, fatigue, headache • The change from mood elevation to mood depression is particularly rapid (< 1 hr) with use of cocaine.
Hallucinogens • Marijuana • Hashish • LSD • PCP • Psilocybin • Mescaline	• Mood elevation, altered perception, hallucinations, bad trips, "flashbacks," cardiovascular symptoms, sweating, tremor • Nystagmus (abnormal eye movements) and episodes of violent behavior and convulsions with PCP	• Few if any withdrawal symptoms

LSD = lysergic acid diethylamide; PCP = phencyclidine.

III. TREATMENT

Clinical snapshot 6-2. A 45-year-old man goes to his physician for a physical examination to obtain a life insurance policy. Although he is a smoker, when filling out his patient information form he checks the box marked "Never smoked." He is denied the policy when the insurance company analyzes his urine sample and finds evidence that he is a smoker.

What evidence has the laboratory found? (see Table 6-3)

A. Laboratory findings can often confirm substance use (Table 6-3).

Table 6-3
Laboratory Findings for Selected Drugs of Abuse

Class of Substance	Elevated Levels in Body Fluids (e.g., urine, blood)	Substance Detection (Length of Time After Use)
Sedatives	• Alcohol: Legal intoxication is 0.08%–0.15% blood alcohol concentration (BAC), depending on state laws. Coma occurs at BAC of 0.40%–0.50% in nonalcoholics.	Within hours
	• Gamma-glutamyltransferase (GGT)	Within hours after alcohol use
	• Specific barbiturate or benzodiazepine or its metabolite	7 days or less
Opioids	• Opiate other than methadone	12–36 hours
	• Methadone	2–3 days
Stimulants	• Cotinine (nicotine metabolite)	1–2 days
	• Amphetamine	1–2 days
	• Benzoylecgonine (cocaine metabolite)	1–3 days in occasional users; 7–12 days in heavy users
Hallucinogens	• Cannabinoid metabolites	7–28 days
	• PCP: Serum glutamic-oxaloacetic transaminase (SGOT) and creatinine phosphokinase (CPK)	More than 7 days

Table 6-4
Treatment for Substance Abuse*

Substance	Treatment
Alcohol	• Alcoholics Anonymous (AA) or other peer support group (12-step program), which are the most effective treatments in the long term • Disulfiram (Antabuse), which causes a toxic reaction when alcohol is ingested; effective to prevent use in motivated patients • Thiamine (Vitamin B$_1$), which is used for emergency room treatment of intoxication • Benzodiazepines (e.g., chlordiazepoxide, diazepam), which are used for withdrawal symptoms
Heroin	• Methadone and LAMM maintenance programs: Both suppress heroin withdrawal symptoms, have a longer duration of action and less sedating and euphoric effects than heroin, are legally dispensed by federal health authorities and can be taken orally; methadone and LAMM cause physical dependence and tolerance. • Naloxone, which blocks opiate receptors, can be used to maintain abstinence. • Clonidine, which stabilizes the autonomic nervous system, is useful for withdrawal symptoms.
Nicotine (cigarette smoking)	• Most abstainers relapse within 2 years; fewer relapse if members of a peer support group. • Antidepressants, particularly bupropion [Zyban], are effective when used as part of a smoking cessation program.

LAMM = l-alpha-acetylmethadol acetate.
* Listed in order of highest to lowest utility

B. **Treatment of substance abuse** ranges from abstinence and peer support groups to drugs that block withdrawal symptoms (Table 6-4).

C. **Dual diagnosis**—or medically ill, chemically addicted (MICA)—patients require treatment for both substance abuse and comorbid psychiatric illness (e.g., major depression). They are often treated on a special unit in the hospital.

Answers to Patient Snapshot Questions

6-1. The substance most likely to be responsible for this man's behavior is cocaine. Cocaine works quickly to elevate mood. However, withdrawal is associated in a short period of time with mood depression.

6-2. Cotinine, a metabolite of nicotine, is the evidence that the laboratory has found in the urine of this patient.

7
Sleep

I. THE AWAKE STATE AND THE NORMAL SLEEP STATE

 Patient snapshot 7-1. The sleep architecture of a patient in a sleep laboratory shows a short REM latency, reduced delta sleep and nine nighttime awakenings. **What psychiatric diagnosis is associated with this sleep pattern?** (see I C 1 b)

A. Awake state. Beta and alpha waves characterize the electroencephalogram (EEG) of an awake individual (Table 7-1).

B. Sleep state. Normal sleep consists of stages 1, 2, 3, and 4 as well as rapid eye movement (REM) sleep. Each stage of sleep is associated with particular brain wave patterns (see Table 7-1).

C. Sleep architecture. The changes in sleep stages that occur throughout the night produce a structure known as sleep architecture.

   1. Sleep architecture changes with age and in depression (Figure 7-1).
   a. In **aging,** sleep is characterized by **repeated nighttime awakenings, reduced slow-wave sleep,** and **reduced REM sleep.**
   b. In **major depressive disorder,** sleep is characterized by normal sleep onset, repeated nighttime awakenings, and **waking too early in the morning.** Short REM latency, long first REM period, and reduced slow-wave sleep also occur.

   2. Use of **alcohol, benzodiazepines,** and **barbiturates** is associated with decreased REM and delta sleep.

D. Neurotransmitters are associated with the production of sleep (Table 7-2).

II. SLEEP DISORDERS

A. Classification of sleep disorders. Many people suffer from sleep disorders. According to the *Diagnostic and Statistical Manual of Mental Disorders*, 4th edition (**DSM-IV**), there are two major categories of sleep disorders:

   1. Dyssomnias are characterized by problems in the timing, quality, or amount of sleep. These disorders include insomnia, narcolepsy, breathing-related sleep disorder (sleep apnea) [Table 7-3], as well as circadian rhythm sleep disorder (sleeping at the inappropriate times) and hypersomnia (oversleeping).

   2. Parasomnias are characterized by abnormalities in physiology or in behavior associated with sleep. They include sleep terror disorder (see Table 7-3), sleepwalking, and nightmare disorders.

Table 7-1
Characteristics of the Awake State and of Sleep Stages

Sleep Stage	Associated EEG Pattern	% Sleep Time in Young Adults	Characteristics
Awake	Beta Alpha	— —	Active mental concentration Relaxation with eyes closed
Stage 1	Theta	5%	Lightest stage of sleep characterized by peacefulness, slowed pulse and respiration, decreased blood pressure, and episodic body movements
Stage 2	Sleep spindle and K-complex	45%	Largest percentage of sleep time
Stages 3 and 4	Delta (slow-wave sleep)	25% (decreases with age)	Deepest, most relaxed stage of sleep; sleep disorders, such as night terrors, sleepwalking (somnambulism), and bed-wetting (enuresis) may occur
Rapid eye movement (REM) sleep	"Sawtooth", beta, alpha, and theta	25% (decreases with age)	Periods occur every 90 min; dreaming; penile and clitoral erection; increased cardiovascular activity; absence of skeletal muscle movement; REM deprivation leads to REM "rebound" and transient psychiatric symptoms

Adapted from Fadem B: *BRS Behavioral Science,* 3e. Philadelphia, Lippincott, Williams and Wilkins, 2000, p. 88.

B. Treatment of sleep disorders. Treatment options for insomnia, narcolepsy, sleep apnea, and sleep terror disorder are described in Table 7-3.

Answer to Patient Snapshot Question

7-1. The sleep architecture of this patient is associated with depression. Sleep in depression is characterized by a short REM latency, reduced delta (slow-wave) sleep, and repeated nighttime awakenings. The patient snapshots in Table 7-3 are explained in the text of the table.

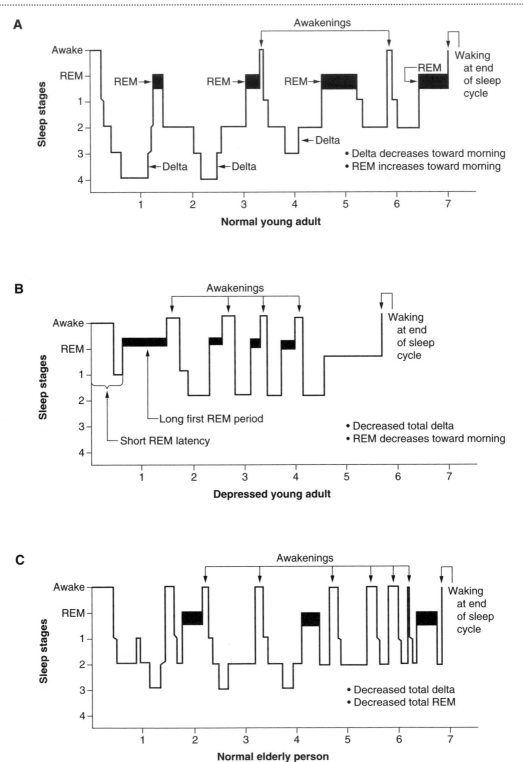

Figure 7-1. Sleep architecture in normal young adults, depressed young adults, and normal elderly persons. REM = rapid eye movement. (Adapted from Wedding D: *Behavior and Medicine*. St. Louis, Mosby Year Book, 1995, p. 416.)

Table 7-2
Neurotransmitters and Sleep

Action	Neurotransmitter	Specific Effect
Promote Sleep	Serotonin	• Increases total sleep time and slow-wave sleep; damage to the dorsal raphe nucleus decreases both of these measures. • Depression is associated with low serotonin, and reduced sleep quality and slow-wave sleep.
	Acetylcholine (Ach)	• Activity in the reticular formation increases total sleep time and REM sleep. ACH levels, total sleep time, and REM sleep decrease in normal aging as well as in Alzheimer disease.
Promote Wakefulness	Norepinephrine	• Decreases both total sleep time and REM sleep • Anxious patients have trouble falling asleep.
	Dopamine (DA)	• Mania and other psychotic illnesses are associated with poor sleep. • Treatment with antipsychotics, which block dopamine receptors, improves sleep.

REM = rapid eye movement.

Table 7-3
Sleep Disorders and Their Treatment

Disorder	Patient Snapshot	Characteristic	Treatment
Insomnia	A 25-year-old medical student complains that for the past year he lies awake in bed for 2 hours before falling asleep at night. During the day, he is tired and makes errors in school.	• Difficulty falling asleep or staying asleep that occurs 3 times weekly for at least 1 month and leads to sleepiness during the day or results in problems fulfilling social or occupational obligations • Occurs in 30% of the United States population • Associated with excessive caffeine intake, anxiety, and mood disorders	• Avoidance of caffeine • Development of a sleep ritual • Fixed sleep and wake schedule • Relaxation techniques
Narcolepsy	A 30-year-old woman reports strange perceptual experiences as she is falling asleep.	• Sleep "attacks" in which the individual falls asleep suddenly during the day • Short REM latency	• Stimulant drugs, such as methylphenidate (Ritalin); if cataplexy is present, antidepressants are added

(continued)

Table 7-3—*Continued*
Sleep Disorders and Their Treatment

Disorder	Patient Snapshot	Characteristic	Treatment
Narcolepsy *(cont.)*	She also has had a few car accidents caused by her falling asleep while driving.	• Hypnagogic hallucinations (occur on falling asleep) • Hypnopompic hallucinations (occur on waking up) • Cataplexy (loss of all muscle tone with a strong emotional stimulus) • Sleep paralysis (inability to move for a few seconds on waking) • Most common in adolescents and young adults	• Timed daytime naps
Breathing related sleep disorder (sleep apnea)	A 45-year-old overweight man is tired every day. His wife reports that he snores and seems to stop breathing at times during the night.	• Breathing cessation for a brief period of time during sleep • It may be central, (no respiratory effort) or obstructive (airway obstruction; is more common) • Cannot sleep deeply because anoxia causes awakenings during the night, leading to chronic tiredness • More common in men, in middle age, and in the obese • Related to headaches, pulmonary hypertension, depression, and sudden death (particularly in the elderly and in infants)	• Weight loss • A device providing continuous positive airway pressure (CPAP) • Surgery (e.g. tracheostomy) as a last resort
Sleep terror disorder	A 4-year-old girl's parents report that she often screams in her sleep during the night. When they try to waken her, she does not respond and has no memory of the incident the next day.	• Nighttime periods of terror • Most common in children • Related to enuresis and sleepwalking • Occurs during slow-wave sleep • No memory of arousal or dreaming • May be an early sign of temporal lobe epilepsy	• Counseling to parents • Reduce stressful family situations • Rarely, use of diazepam in small doses at bedtime

*In order of highest to lowest utility

8

The Genetics of Behavior

I. GENETIC STUDIES

A. **Pedigree studies** use a **family tree** to show the occurrence of traits and diseases within a family.

B. **Family risk studies** compare how frequently a disease occurs in the relatives of the affected individual (**proband**) with how frequently it occurs in the general population.

C. Twin studies

   1. **Adoption studies** using **monozygotic twins** (who are derived from a single fertilized ovum) or **dizygotic twins** (who are derived from two fertilized ova), reared together or apart, are used to distinguish the effects of genetic factors from environmental factors in disease.

   2. If both twins have a given trait, they are **concordant** for that trait.

   3. If genetic in origin, a disorder may be expected to occur more often in monozygotic twins than in dizygotic twins.

II. GENETIC ORIGINS OF PSYCHIATRIC DISORDERS

 Patient snapshot 8-1. A 22-year-old woman reports that she just learned that her father—whom she believed had died when she was an infant—has been institutionalized for the last 20 years suffering from schizophrenia.

What are the chances that this woman will develop schizophrenia over the course of her life? (see Table 8-1)

A. Schizophrenia (see Chapter 11)

   1. **Prevalence.** The prevalence of schizophrenia is about **1%** in the general population. The prevalence is approximately **equal in men and women,** with no ethnic differences in its occurrence.

   2. Persons with a **close genetic relationship** to an individual with schizophrenia are more likely than those with a more distant relationship to be concordant for, or to develop, the disorder (Table 8-1).

   3. **Genetic markers** on **chromosomes 1, 6, 8 and 13** have been associated with schizophrenia.

B. Affective (mood) disorders (see Chapter 12)

   1. Prevalence

Table 8-1
Risk of Developing Schizophrenia and Bipolar Disorder in Relatives of Patients

Group	Risk for Schizophrenia (%)	Risk for Bipolar Disorder (%)
First-degree relative of a person (sibling, dizygotic twin, parent) with the disorder	10	20
Child who has two parents with the disorder	40	60
Monozygotic twin of a person with the disorder	50	75

    a. The lifetime prevalence of major depressive disorder is about **10% in men** and **15% to 20% in women.**

    b. The **lifetime prevalence** of bipolar disorder is about **1%** with no gender differences in its occurrence.

  2. The **genetic component is stronger in bipolar disorder** than in major depressive disorder or schizophrenia (see Table 8-1).

  3. No specific genetic markers have been identified in the etiology of the affective disorders.

C. **Personality characteristics and disorders** (see Chapter 14)

  1. Personality characteristics, such as responsiveness to stimulation, fearfulness, activity level, and distractibility, have a higher concordance rate in monozygotic twins than in dizygotic twins.

  2. **Genetic factors** also play a role in personality disorders. Relatives of patients with specific personality disorders have demonstrated characteristic psychiatric problems (Table 8-2).

III. GENETIC ORIGINS OF NEUROPSYCHIATRIC DISORDERS

 Patient snapshot 8-2. Physical examination of a 48-year-old woman with the symptoms of Alzheimer disease reveals that she has midface depression, extra skin at the corners of her eyes, and an enlarged tongue.

Which chromosome is most likely involved in this patient's problem? (see III A 2)

A. **Alzheimer disease** is a progressive deterioration of cognitive functioning. In many cases, there is a **family history** of the disease.

Table 8-2
Psychiatric Conditions Observed in Relatives of Patients with Personality Disorders*

Personality Disorder of Patient	Psychiatric Condition Seen in Relatives
Antisocial	Alcoholism; ADHD
Avoidant	Anxiety disorders
Borderline	Major depressive disorder; substance abuse
Histrionic	Somatization disorder
Schizotypal	Schizophrenia

ADHD = attention deficit hyperactivity disorder.
*See Chapters 11, 12, and 14

1. **Twin studies.** There is a higher concordance rate for Alzheimer disease in monozygotic twins than that in dizygotic twins.

2. **Chromosome 21**
   a. This chromosome, which is associated with **Down syndrome,** has been found to be defective in some patients with Alzheimer disease.
   b. Individuals with Down syndrome who live beyond 40 years of age develop symptoms resembling Alzheimer disease.

3. **Chromosomes 1 and 14.** Recently, these chromosomes have been implicated in Alzheimer disease, particularly in the type with an early onset (before age 65 years).

4. The **apolipoprotein E4 (apo E4) gene** on chromosome 19 also has been implicated in Alzheimer disease.

B. **Other neuropsychiatric disorders** and forms of mental retardation with genetic components include:

1. **Huntington disease,** in which there is an abnormal gene on the short end of chromosome 4

2. **Down and fragile X syndromes,** which are the first and second most common genetic causes of mental retardation, respectively

3. **Lesch-Nyhan syndrome,** in which there is X-linked transmission

4. **Tourette disorder,** in which 90% of patients have a family member who is also affected

IV. ALCOHOLISM

A. **Prevalence.** Alcoholism is **four times more prevalent** in children of alcoholics than in children of nonalcoholics, even if the children are raised by adoptive parents.

B. The **concordance rate** for alcoholism is 60% in monozygotic twins and 30% in dizygotic twins.

C. **Family history. Sons of alcoholics** are at **greater risk than daughters** of alcoholics. The genetic influence is strongest in males who abuse alcohol before 20 years of age.

Answers to Patient Snapshot Questions

8-1. The chances that this woman, whose father is schizophrenic, will develop the illness is approximately 10%.
8-2. The physical description of this patient indicates that she has Down syndrome. Chromosome 21 is involved in the etiology of Down syndrome and Alzheimer disease.

9

Behavioral Neurochemistry

I. NEUROANATOMY

 Patient snapshot 9-1. A 48-year-old male patient shows increased emotionality following a stroke.

What area of his brain is most likely to have been affected by the stroke? (see Table 9-1)

A. The **central nervous system (CNS)** contains the brain and spinal cord.

  1. The cerebral hemispheres of the brain are connected by the corpus callosum, anterior commissure, hippocampal commissure, posterior commissure, and habenular commissure.

  2. The **functions** of the hemispheres are **lateralized.**
   a. The **right,** or **nondominant, hemisphere** is associated primarily with **perception;** it also is associated with **spatial relations** and musical and artistic ability.
   b. The **left,** or **dominant, hemisphere** is associated with **language function** in about 96% of right-handed persons and 70% of left-handed persons.

B. The **peripheral nervous system (PNS)** contains all sensory, motor, and autonomic fibers outside of the CNS, including the spinal nerves, cranial nerves, and peripheral ganglia.

  1. The PNS carries sensory information to the CNS and motor information away from the CNS.

  2. The **autonomic nervous system,** which consists of sympathetic and parasympathetic divisions, innervates the internal organs.
   a. This system coordinates emotional experiences with visceral responses (e.g., changes in heart rate or blood pressure).
   b. Visceral responses occurring as a result of psychological stress are involved in the exacerbation of some physical illnesses (see Chapter 20).

C. **Brain lesions** caused by accident, disease, or surgery are associated with particular neuropsychiatric deficits (Table 9-1).

II. NEUROTRANSMISSION

A. Synapses and neurotransmitters

  1. When the presynaptic neuron is stimulated, a **neurotransmitter** is released, travels across the synaptic cleft, and acts on receptors on the postsynaptic neuron.

Table 9-1
Neuropsychiatric Effects of Brain Lesions

Location of Lesion	Effects
Frontal lobes	• Emotional symptoms (e.g., depression, especially with dominant lesions) • Problems with attention, motivation, concentration, and orientation
Parietal lobes	• Impaired processing of visual-spatial (right-sided lesions) information and verbal (left-sided lesions) information
Temporal lobes Limbic system Hypothalamus	• Impaired memory • Hallucinations • Personality changes • Poor new learning (hippocampus) • Decreased aggressive behavior, increased sexual behavior, and hyperorality (Klüver-Bucy syndrome) (amygdala) • Decreased fear response (amygdala) • Increased appetite leading to obesity (ventromedial nucleus [satiety center] damage) • Loss of appetite leading to weight loss (lateral nucleus damage) • Effects on sexual activity and body temperature regulation
Reticular system	• Changes in sleep-wake mechanisms (e.g., increased production of REM sleep via increased acetylcholine production)
Basal ganglia	• Disorders of movement, such as Parkinson disease (substantia nigra), Huntington disease (caudate and putamen), and Tourette syndrome (caudate)

2. Neurotransmitters are **excitatory** if they increase the chances that a neuron will fire and **inhibitory** if they decrease these chances.

B. **Presynaptic and postsynaptic receptors** are proteins present in the membrane of the neuron that can recognize specific neurotransmitters.

  1. The **changeability** of number or affinity of receptors for specific neurotransmitters (**neuronal plasticity**) can regulate the responsiveness of neurons.

  2. **Second messengers.** When stimulated by neurotransmitters, postsynaptic receptors may alter the metabolism of the neuron by the use of second messengers, which include **cyclic adenosine monophosphate (cAMP), lipids** (e.g., diacylglycerol), and Ca^{2+}.

C. **Classification.** The three major classes of neurotransmitters are **biogenic amines** (monoamines), **amino acids,** and **peptides.**

D. Regulation of neurotransmitter activity

  1. The concentration of neurotransmitters in the synaptic cleft is closely related to mood and behavior. A number of mechanisms affect this concentration.

   a. After release by the presynaptic neuron, neurotransmitters are removed from the synaptic cleft by **reuptake** by the presynaptic neuron.

   b. Neurotransmitters may also be **degraded by enzymes,** such as **monoamine oxidase (MAO).**

    2. Availability of specific neurotransmitters is associated with the etiology of many psychiatric conditions (Table 9-2).

        a. Normalization of neurotransmitter levels by pharmacologic agents can ameliorate many of the symptoms of these disorders.

        b. Mechanisms by which these agents work include blocking reuptake of neurotransmitters and blocking the enzymes that degrade them.

III. BIOGENIC AMINES

 Patient snapshot 9-2. A 30-year-old man is brought to the emergency department with a serious knife wound to the chest. The wound is a result of a fight that the patient started when another man refused to give up a parking space.

The body fluids of this assaultive, impulsive patient are most likely to show decreased levels of the major metabolite of which neurotransmitter? (see Table 9-3)

A. Overview

    1. The **biogenic amines,** or **monoamines,** include catecholamines, indolamines, ethylamines, and quaternary amines.

    2. The **monoamine theory of mood disorder** hypothesizes that **lowered noradrenergic or serotonergic activity results in depression.**

    3. Metabolites of the monoamines are measured in psychiatric research and diagnosis because they are present in body fluids at higher levels than the actual monoamines (Table 9-3).

B. Dopamine

    1. Dopamine, a catecholamine, is involved in the pathophysiology of **schizophrenia, Parkinson disease,** and **mood disorders.**

    2. Synthesis. The amino acid tyrosine is converted to the precursor for dopamine by the action of **tyrosine hydroxylase.**

C. Norepinephrine, a catecholamine, plays a role in **mood, anxiety, arousal, and learning and memory.**

    1. Synthesis

        a. Like dopaminergic neurons, noradrenergic neurons synthesize dopamine.

        b. β-hydroxylase, present in noradrenergic neurons, converts dopamine to norepinephrine.

    2. Localization. Most noradrenergic neurons (approximately 10,000 per hemisphere in the brain) are located in the **locus ceruleus.**

Table 9-2
Psychiatric Conditions and Associated Neurotransmitter Activity

Psychiatric Condition	Neurotransmitter Activity Increased ($\uparrow$) or Decreased ($\downarrow$)
Schizophrenia	Dopamine ($\uparrow$), serotonin ($\uparrow$)
Mania	Dopamine ($\uparrow$)
Depression	Norepinephrine ($\downarrow$), serotonin ($\downarrow$), dopamine ($\downarrow$)
Anxiety	GABA ($\downarrow$), serotonin ($\downarrow$), norepinephrine ($\uparrow$)
Alzheimer disease	Acetylcholine ($\downarrow$)

GABA = γ-aminobutyric acid.

Table 9-3
Metabolites of Monoamines and Associated Psychopathology

Neurotransmitter	Concentration of Metabolite*	Associated Psychopathology
Dopamine	Increased HVA	• Schizophrenia • Other conditions involving psychosis
	Decreased HVA	• Parkinson disease • Depression • Alcoholism
Norepinephrine	Decreased MHPG	• Severe depression
	Increased VMA	• Adrenal medulla tumor (pheochromocytoma)
Serotonin	Decreased 5-HIAA	• Severe depression • Violent behavior • Impulsive behavior • Fire setting • Tourette syndrome • Alcohol abuse • Bulimia

5-HIAA = 5-hydroxyindoleacetic acid; HVA = homovanillic acid; MHPG = 3-methoxy-4-hydroxyphenylglycol; VMA = vanillylmandelic acid.
*In blood plasma, cerebrospinal fluid, or urine.

D. Serotonin, an indolamine, plays a role in **mood, sexuality, sleep, and impulse control;** high levels of serotonin are associated with **improved mood and sleep** but **decreased sexual functioning** (see Chapter 18). Decreased serotonin is associated with depression, poor impulse control, and poor sleep.

  1. Synthesis. The amino acid tryptophan is converted to serotonin, also known as **5-hydroxytryptamine (5-HT),** by the enzyme tryptophan hydroxylase as well as by an amino acid decarboxylase.

  2. Localization. Most serotonergic cell bodies in the brain are contained in the **dorsal raphe nucleus.**

  3. Antidepressant agents (see Chapter 10) ultimately increase the presence of serotonin (and sometimes also of norepinephrine) in the synaptic cleft; the selective serotonin reuptake inhibitors (SSRIs), such as **fluoxetine (Prozac),** work specifically by **blocking the reuptake** of serotonin into the presynaptic neuron.

E. Histamine

  1. Histamine, an **ethylamine,** is affected by psychoactive agents.

  2. Histamine receptor blockade by agents such as antipsychotics and tricyclic antidepressants is associated with common side effects, such as sedation and increased appetite (leading to weight gain).

F. Acetylcholine (ACh), a quaternary amine, is the transmitter used by **nerve-skeleton-muscle junctions.**

  1. Degeneration of cholinergic neurons is associated with **Alzheimer disease, Down syndrome,** and **movement and sleep disorders.**

  2. Synthesis and breakdown of ACh

   a. **Cholinergic neurons** synthesize ACh from acetyl coenzyme A and choline using **choline acetyltransferase.**

   b. **Acetylcholinesterase** (AChE) breaks ACh down into choline and acetate; blocking the action of AChE with drugs such as tacrine (Cognex) and donepezil (Aricept) can delay the progression of Alzheimer disease but cannot reverse lost function.

IV. AMINO ACID NEUROTRANSMITTERS are involved in most synapses in the brain. These neurotransmitters include γ-aminobutyric acid (GABA), glycine, and glutamate.

A. **GABA** is the principal inhibitory neurotransmitter in the CNS and is involved in the antianxiety activity of the benzodiazepines and barbiturates.

B. **Glycine** is an inhibitory neurotransmitter that acts independently and also as a regulator of glutamate activity.

C. **Glutamate** is an excitatory neurotransmitter and may be associated with **epilepsy, neurodegenerative illnesses,** and **mechanisms of cell death.**

V. NEUROPEPTIDES

A. **Endogenous opioids**

   1. **Enkephalins** and **endorphins** are endogenous opioids that affect pain, thermoregulation, seizure activity, anxiety, and mood.

   2. **Placebo effects** may be mediated by the endogenous opioid system and may be blocked by treatment with an opiate receptor blocker such as naloxone.

B. **Other neuropeptides** have been implicated in the following conditions.

   1. **Schizophrenia** [cholecystokinin (CCK) and neurotensin]

   2. **Mood disorders** [somatostatin, substance P, vasopressin, oxytocin, and vasoactive intestinal peptide (VIP)]

   3. **Pain and aggression** (substance P)

   4. **Alzheimer disease** (somatostatin and VIP)

Answers to Patient Snapshot Questions

9-1. The brain areas most closely involved in emotion are the frontal lobes.

9-2. Decreased levels of brain serotonin are most closely involved in impulsive, aggressive, assaultive behavior. The major metabolite of serotonin, 5-hydroxyindoleacetic acid, would therefore be decreased in this man.

10

Pharmacology of Behavior and Electroconvulsive Therapy

I. AGENTS USED TO TREAT PSYCHOSIS

 Patient snapshot 10-1. A 40-year-old woman with chronic schizophrenia has been taking an antipsychotic medication for 6 years. Recently, she has begun to show involuntary lip smacking and chewing movements of her mouth and tongue.

What type of antipsychotic agent has this patient been taking, and what action should the physician take? (see Tables 10-1 and 10-2)

A. **Traditional, or typical, antipsychotic agents**

1. Traditional antipsychotics are used to treat **schizophrenia** and psychosis associated with other psychiatric and physical disorders (see Chapter 11).

2. Their primary mechanism of action is as D_2 receptor antagonists and they are classified according to **potency.**
    a. **Low-potency agents** are associated primarily with anticholinergic, endocrine, hematologic, dermatologic, ophthalmologic, and antihistaminergic side effects.

Table 10-1
Neurologic Adverse Effects of Traditional High-Potency Antipsychotics and Their Treatment

Effects	Characteristics
Extrapyramidal effects	• Pseudoparkinsonism (muscle rigidity, shuffling gait, resting tremor, mask-like facial expression) • Akathisia (subjective feeling of motor restlessness) • Acute dystonia (prolonged muscular spasms); more common in men younger than age 40 • Treat with an anticholinergic (e.g., benztropine) or antihistaminergic (e.g., diphenhydramine) agent
Other effects	• Tardive dyskinesia (abnormal writhing movements of the tongue, face, and body); more common in women and after at least 6 months of treatment • Treat by substituting with a low-potency or atypical antipsychotic agent • Neuroleptic malignant syndrome (high fever, sweating, increased pulse and blood pressure, muscular rigidity); more common in men and early in treatment; mortality rate about 20% • Decreased seizure threshold • Treat by discontinuing agent and providing medical support

Table 10-2
Traditional and Atypical Antipsychotic Agents

Type of Agent and Specific Agents	Advantages	Disadvantages
Traditional high-potency agents • Haloperidol (Haldol) • Perphenazine (Trilafon) • Trifluoperazine (Stelazine)	• Positive symptoms improve in about 70% of patients.	• More neurologic adverse effects than low-potency agents • Less effective against negative symptoms than atypical agents
Traditional low-potency agents • Chlorpromazine (Thorazine) • Thioridazine (Mellaril)	• Fewer neurological adverse effects than high-potency agents	• More nonneurologic adverse effects (ie, anticholinergic effects) than high-potency agents • Less effective against negative symptoms than atypical agents
Atypical agents • Clozapine (Clozaril) • Risperidone (Risperdal) • Olanzapine (Zyprexa) • Quetiapine (Seroquel)	• More effective than traditional agents against negative symptoms • Fewer neurologic adverse effects than traditional agents	• More hematologic problems (agranulocytosis), anticholinergic effects, and seizures than traditional agents

    b. **High-potency agents** are associated primarily with neurologic side effects (Table 10-1).

  B. **Atypical antipsychotic agents** are newer drugs that work by a different mechanism of action (i.e., as 5-HT_2 and D_4 receptor antagonists).

    1. They are used to treat psychotic symptoms in patients who are resistant to treatment or unable to tolerate the adverse effects of traditional agents.

    2. These agents have advantages and disadvantages when compared with high- and low-potency traditional agents (Table 10-2).

II. AGENTS USED TO TREAT MOOD DISORDERS

Patient snapshot 10-2. A 45-year-old woman is brought to the emergency department with a severe headache, vomiting, and sweating. Clinical examination reveals greatly elevated blood pressure and a fever. The woman's husband notes that they had just finished eating dinner (which included cheese and red wine) in a French restaurant when her symptoms started.

What class of psychoactive agents is most likely to be responsible for this woman's symptoms? (see II A 3)

  A. Antidepressants

    1. Classification

      a. **Heterocyclic antidepressants** (tricyclic and tetracyclic), **monoamine oxidase (MAO) inhibitors, selective serotonin reuptake inhibitors (SSRIs),** and other antidepressants are used to treat depression (see Chapter 12) as well as other psychiatric disorders (Table 10-3).

        1) All antidepressants take **3–6 weeks for the therapeutic effect** to begin and **all have equal efficacy.**

        2) Antidepressants do not elevate mood in nondepressed people and **have no abuse potential.**

Table 10-3
Antidepressant Agents

Agent	Effects and Clinical Uses
Heterocyclic Agents (HCAs)	
Amitriptyline (Elavil)	• Sedating • Has anticholinergic effects
Clomipramine (Anafranil)	• Most serotonin-specific of the HCAs • Useful to treat obsessive compulsive disorder (OCD)
Desipramine (Norpramin, Pertofrane)	• Least sedating and least anticholinergic of the HCAs • Stimulates appetite • Useful for depression in the elderly
Doxepin (Adapin, Sinequan)	• Sedating • Has antihistaminic and anticholinergic effects
Imipramine (Tofranil)	• Likely to cause orthostatic hypotension • Used to treat enuresis
Nortriptyline (Aventyl, Pamelor)	• Least likely HCA to cause orthostatic hypotension • First choice HCA for depression in the elderly
Selective Serotonin Reuptake Inhibitors (SSRIs)	
Fluoxetine (Prozac, Sarafem)	• May cause agitation, insomnia, and weight loss initially • Sarafem useful for premenstrual syndrome
Fluvoxamine (Luvox)	• Currently indicated only for OCD
Paroxetine (Paxil)	• Most serotonin-specific of the SSRIs
Sertraline (Zoloft)	• The most likely SSRI to cause gastrointestinal disturbances (e.g., diarrhea)
Citalopram (Celexa)	• The newest SSRI
Monoamine Oxidase Inhibitors (MAOIs)	
Isocarboxazid (Marplan) Phenelzine (Nardil) Tranylcypromine (Parnate)	• All MAOIs are useful for atypical depression, panic disorder, eating disorders, pain disorders • Social phobia (phenelzine) • Dietary precautions are necessary with all MAOIs (see text)
Other Antidepressants	
Amoxapine (Asendin)	• Antidopaminergic effects such as pseudoparkinsonism • Useful for depression with psychotic features • Dangerous in overdose
Bupropion (Wellbutrin, Zyban)	• Insomnia, seizures, sweating • Fewer adverse sexual effects • Zyban used for smoking cessation
Mirtazepine (Remeron)	• Targets specific serotonin receptors • Few side effects
Nefazodone (Serzone)	• Related to trazodone, but has fewer side effects
Trazodone (Desyrel)	• Sedating • Causes priapism (persistent erection) • Safe in overdose
Venlafaxine (Effexor)	• Serotonergic and noradrenergic effects • Low cytochrome P_{450} effects

    b. **Stimulants,** such as methylphenidate or dextroamphetamine, may also be useful in treating depression, particularly in the elderly or terminally ill. Disadvantages include their addiction potential.

2. Heterocyclics
    a. Heterocyclic agents **block the reuptake of norepinephrine and serotonin** at the synapse, increasing the availability of these neurotransmitters and improving mood.
    b. These agents also block muscarinic acetylcholine and histamine receptors, causing **anticholinergic effects, sedation,** and **weight gain.** An **overdose may be fatal.**

3. MAO inhibitors
    a. MAO inhibitors irreversibly limit the action of MAO, **increasing the availability of norepinephrine and serotonin** in the synaptic cleft and improving mood.
    b. MAO inhibitors may be particularly useful in treating **atypical depression** (see Chapter 12) and treatment resistance to other agents.
    c. Because **MAO metabolizes tyramine,** a pressor, in the gastrointestinal tract, the ingestion of tyramine-rich foods (e.g., aged cheese, beer, wine, broad beans, chicken or beef liver, orange pulp, smoked or pickled meats or fish) or sympathomimetic agents (e.g., pseudoephedrine [Sudafed]) can lead to a **hypertensive crisis, which may result in stroke or death.**
    d. MAO inhibitors are as safe as heterocyclics if **dietary precautions** are followed. Adverse effects are similar to those of the heterocyclics.

4. SSRIs
    a. SSRIs selectively **block the reuptake of serotonin,** but have little effect on dopamine, norepinephrine, histamine, or acetylcholine systems.
    b. Compared with heterocyclic antidepressants, SSRIs are equivalent in efficacy, have **minimal anticholinergic and cardiovascular adverse effects, do not cause sedation, and may cause weight loss.**
    c. SSRIs are now used as **first-line agents for depression.** When compared with other antidepressants, the SSRIs are safer for the elderly and for pregnant women.
    d. The SSRIs are also useful in the treatment of **obsessive compulsive disorder, panic disorder,** and **premenstrual syndrome.**
    e. Because they cause sexual dysfunction, including delayed orgasm and ejaculation, they are being used to **treat premature ejaculation.**

B. Mood stabilizers: agents used to treat mania

    1. **Lithium carbonate and lithium citrate** are used primarily to **treat the mania of bipolar disorder.** They also have antidepressant activity.
        a. Adverse effects include renal dysfunction, cardiac conduction abnormalities, gastric distress, tremor, mild cognitive impairment, hypothyroidism, and **first-trimester congenital abnormalities,** especially of the cardiovascular system.
        b. Lithium **takes 2–3 weeks for the therapeutic effect** to begin. **Haloperidol,** which works within hours, is therefore the initial treatment for psychotic symptoms in an acute manic episode.

    2. **Anticonvulsants,** such as **carbamazepine (Tegretol)** and **valproic acid (Depakene, Depakote),** are also used to treat bipolar disorder, particularly **rapid cycling bipolar disorder,** which is characterized by more than 4 episodes annually.

III. ANTIANXIETY AGENTS

Patient snapshot 10-3. A physician needs to choose an antianxiety agent for a 45-year-old man with a history of generalized anxiety disorder and substance abuse.

    Which agent would best relieve the patient's anxiety but have a low risk of abuse? (see III B 1)

A. Benzodiazepines and barbiturates

   1. Benzodiazepines relieve the symptoms of anxiety and can be **short-, intermediate-, or long-acting.** These agents are also used in the management of seizures, for muscle relaxation, and in the treatment of alcohol withdrawal (Table 10-4).

   2. **Tolerance and dependence** occur with chronic use of these agents. Barbiturates have a **greater potential for abuse and a lower therapeutic index** (i.e., the ratio of minimum toxic dose to maximum effective dose) than benzodiazepines.

B. Nonbenzodiazepines

   1. **Buspirone (BuSpar),** an azaspirodecanedione, is unrelated to the benzodiazepines and is **nonsedating.** In contrast to the benzodiazepines, it is **not associated with dependence, abuse, or withdrawal.** It takes up to 2 weeks for the therapeutic effect to begin.

   2. **Zolpidem tartrate (Ambien)** is a short-acting agent unrelated to the benzodiazepines and used primarily **to treat insomnia.**

IV. ELECTROCONVULSIVE THERAPY

A. Uses

   1. Electroconvulsive therapy (ECT) involves inducing a generalized seizure by passing an electric current across the brain. ECT is a safe, effective treatment for **major depressive disorder refractive to other treatment,** the most common indication. It also is effective for treatment of acute mania and schizophrenia with acute, catatonic, or affective symptoms.

   2. The maximum response to ECT usually occurs after **5–10 treatments given over a 2–3 week period.** Biweekly or monthly maintenance ECT may prevent relapse.

Table 10-4
Benzodiazepines

Agent	Duration of Action	Clinical Uses in Addition to Treating Anxiety
Chlorazepate (Tranxene)	Short	Management of partial seizures
Lorazepam (Ativan)	Short	Psychotic agitation, alcohol withdrawal, status epilepticus (persistent seizures)
Oxazepam (Serax)	Short	Alcohol withdrawal
Triazolam (Halcion)	Short	Insomnia
Alprazolam (Xanax)	Intermediate	Depression, panic disorder, social phobia
Temazepam (Restoril)	Intermediate	Insomnia
Chlordiazepoxide (Librium)	Long	First-line agent for alcohol withdrawal
Clonazepam (Klonopin)	Long	Seizures, mania, social phobia, panic disorder, aggression; adjunctive use with mood stabilizers
Diazepam (Valium)	Long	Muscle relaxation, analgesia, anticonvulsant, seizures associated with alcohol withdrawal
Flurazepam (Dalmane)	Long	Insomnia

    B. Adverse effects

        1. Most adverse affects, such as broken bones, have been eliminated with judicious use of **general anesthesia and muscle relaxants** before treatment. The mortality rate is comparable to that associated with general anesthesia.

        2. The major adverse effect of ECT is **amnesia** for past events. In most patients, amnesia resolves within 6 months after treatment concludes.

        3. ECT is **contraindicated** in patients with **increased intracranial pressure.**

        4. Unilateral electrode placement causes less memory impairment but slower therapeutic responses than bilateral placement.

Answers to Patient Snapshot Questions

10-1. This patient is showing signs of tardive dyskinesia and has probably been taking a high-potency antipsychotic agent. The treatment of this side effect of medication is to substitute a low-potency or atypical agent. Simply discontinuing the medication will cause the symptoms to worsen.

10-2. This patient has probably been taking a monoamine oxidase (MAO) inhibitor. She is experiencing a life-threatening hypertensive crisis caused by ingestion of tyramine, which is present in red wine and aged cheese.

10-3. Because this patient has a history of substance abuse, the best agent to relieve his anxiety is buspirone. In contrast to the benzodiazepines, buspirone is nonaddicting and has a very low risk for abuse.

11

Schizophrenia and Other Psychotic Disorders

Patient snapshot 11-1. A 22-year-old medical student with no history of psychiatric illness tells her friend that she believes that the Dean of the medical school is poisoning her food in the cafeteria. She is alert and oriented but seems anxious and frightened. Her symptoms started 2 weeks ago, when she found out that she had failed the first Anatomy exam.

What is the best diagnosis for this student? (see Table 11-1)

I. OVERVIEW (Table 11-1)

A. Schizophrenia is a chronic mental disorder that is present in about 1% of the population in all countries and ethnic groups studied. The disorder is characterized by:

  1. Periods of psychosis (loss of touch with reality), in which delusions and hallucinations occur

  2. Periods between psychotic episodes (residual phases), in which the person is in touch with reality but shows disturbances in behavior, appearance, speech and affect and has peculiar thinking

B. The occurrence of schizophrenia shows no sex difference but there are sex differences in its presentation.

  1. Schizophrenia often **develops at a younger age in male (15–25 years) than in female (25–35 years) patients.**

  2. Men are less responsive to antipsychotic medication and show more deficits in social and cognitive function than women.

II. ETIOLOGY

A. The following neurological factors occur and may be associated with the etiology of schizophrenia:

  1. Hyperactivity of the **dopaminergic, serotonergic, and noradrenergic systems**

  2. Enlargement of the **lateral and third ventricles** of the brain

  3. Abnormalities of the **frontal lobes**

B. No social or environmental factor causes schizophrenia.

  1. Schizophrenia is diagnosed more often in populations of **low socioeconomic status.**

  2. This increased incidence may be caused by **downward drift** into lower socioeconomic

Table 11-1
Differential Diagnoses of Schizophrenia

Disorder	Characteristics
Schizophrenia	• Psychotic and residual symptoms lasting > 6 months
Brief psychotic disorder	• Psychotic and residual symptoms lasting > 1 day but < 1 month • There are often precipitating stressful psychosocial factors
Schizophreniform disorder	• Psychotic and residual symptoms lasting 1–6 months
Schizoaffective disorder	• Symptoms of a mood disorder as well as schizophrenia • Chronic social and occupational impairment
Manic phase of bipolar disorder	• Psychotic symptoms, elevated mood, hyperactivity, rapid speech, increased sociability • Little or no impairment in social or occupational functioning between episodes
Delusional disorder and shared psychotic disorder	• Fixed, pervasive, non-bizarre delusional system • Few if any other thought disorders • Relatively normal social and occupational functioning in a patient or his close relative (shared psychotic disorder)
Schizoid personality disorder	• Social withdrawal without psychosis
Schizotypal personality disorder	• Peculiar behavior and odd thought patterns, such as magical thinking (i.e., believing that something one wishes can alter the course of events in the world) • No frank psychosis
Borderline personality disorder	• Extreme mood changes with uncontrollable anger and episodic suicidal thoughts • Mini-psychotic episodes (lasting only minutes)
Substance-induced psychotic disorder	• Prominent hallucinations (often visual or tactile) or delusions directly related to use of stimulants or hallucinogens or withdrawal from sedatives (see Chapter 10)
Psychotic disorder due to a general medical condition (delirium)	• Clouding of consciousness • Hallucinations are visual and changeable rather than auditory and recurrent • Occurs in the context of an acute medical illness

Adapted from Fadem B, Simring S: *High-Yield Psychiatry*. Baltimore: Lippincott, Williams and Wilkins, 1998, p. 58.

classes, which occurs because individuals with schizophrenia show decreased social and occupational functioning.

III. CLINICAL SIGNS AND SYMPTOMS

A. Affected individuals show evidence of **disordered thinking** and psychosis. Symptoms include **hallucinations,** most commonly auditory, **bizarre behavior,** and **delusions. Flat, blunted, or inappropriate affect** may also be present.

1. Symptoms must be present for **more than 6 months,** with **impairment of occupational or social functioning.**

2. The patient is usually alert, **oriented to person, place, and time,** and has a **good memory;** if not, a cognitive disorder should be suspected (see Chapter 13).

B. Classification of symptoms. Symptoms can be classified as positive or negative. This classification can be useful in predicting the effects of antipsychotic medication.

   1. Positive symptoms are things additional to expected behavior and include delusions, hallucinations, agitation and talkativeness. Positive symptoms respond well to most **traditional antipsychotic medication.**

   2. Negative symptoms are things missing from expected behavior and include flattening of affect, deficiencies in speech content, poor grooming, lack of motivation, and social withdrawal. Negative symptoms respond better to **atypical agents** than to traditional antipsychotics.

C. Thought disorders

   1. Disorders of content of thought include **delusions and ideas of reference.** A distinction is made between these disorders and hallucinations and illusions that are perceptual disturbances (Table 11-2).

   2. Disorders of form of thought include incoherence, word salad (i.e., using unrelated combination of words), loose associations, neologisms (i.e., using newly invented words), and echolalia (i.e., repeating words).

   3. Disorders of thought processes include flight of ideas (i.e., rapid succession of thoughts), illogical ideas, thought blocking, short attention span, deficiencies in thought and content of speech, impaired memory and abstraction abilities, and clang associations (i.e., speaking in rhyming words).

D. Subtypes and differential diagnosis

   1. Subtypes. The *Diagnostic and Statistical Manual of Mental Disorders,* 4th edition (DSM-IV), lists five subtypes of schizophrenia: disorganized (hebephrenic); catatonic; paranoid; undifferentiated; and residual (Table 11-3).

   2. Other disorders characterized by psychotic symptoms and bizarre behavior (see Table 11-1)

   a. All psychotic disorders are characterized at some point in their course by a **loss**

Table 11-2
Illusions, Hallucinations, Delusions, and Ideas of Reference

Symptom	Definition	Patient Snapshot
Illusion	Misperception of real external stimuli	A man who is alone in a room in the dark thinks that his jacket on the chair is a man.
Hallucination	False sensory perception	A woman who is alone in a room hears a voice outside of her head telling her to jump from the window.
Delusion	False belief not shared by others	A homeless woman tells the physician that she is being followed by government agents.
Idea of reference	False belief of being referred to by others	A man states that a television host is talking about him every morning.

Table 11-3
DSM-IV Subtypes of Schizophrenia

Subtype	Characteristics
Disorganized	Disinhibited, disorganized, disheveled personal appearance, inappropriate emotional response; onset before 25 years of age
Catatonic	Stupor or agitation, lack of coherent speech, bizarre posturing (waxy flexibility); rare since the introduction of antipsychotic agents
Paranoid	Delusions of persecution; better social functioning and older age at onset than other subtypes
Undifferentiated	Characteristics of more than one subtype
Residual	At least one psychotic episode; subsequent flat affect, illogical thinking, odd behavior, and social withdrawal, but no severe psychotic symptoms

DSM-IV = *Diagnostic and Statistical Manual of Mental Disorders,* 4th edition.

of touch with reality (e.g., delusions and/or hallucinations). However, other psychotic disorders do not include all of the criteria required for the diagnosis of schizophrenia.

b. **Differential diagnoses** of schizophrenia include other psychotic disorders such as brief psychotic disorder, schizophreniform disorder, schizoaffective disorder, and delusional disorder.

c. The differential diagnosis also includes the **manic phase of bipolar disorder** (Chapter 12), schizoid and schizotypal **personality disorders** (Chapter 14), and **delirium** (Chapter 13).

IV. PROGNOSIS AND TREATMENT

A. Prognosis

1. Schizophrenia usually involves repeated psychotic episodes and a **chronic downhill course** over years.

2. A **good prognosis** is associated with presence of mood symptoms, female gender, good social and work relationships, positive symptoms, older age at onset, and absence of neurologic symptoms.

3. **Suicide** is common in patients with schizophrenia. More than 50% attempt suicide, and at least 10% of those die in the attempt. **Risk factors** for suicide are male sex, college education, youth, many relapses, depressed mood, high ambitions, and living alone.

B. Treatment

1. **Antipsychotic agents** are the major treatment for schizophrenia (see Chapter 10 I A). Long acting injectable "depot" forms (e.g., haloperidol decanoate) can improve functioning in noncompliant individuals.

2. **Psychosocial interventions,** such as behavioral, family, group, and individual therapy, provide long-term social support and foster compliance with the drug regimen.

Answer to Patient Snapshot Question

11-1. This patient is probably suffering from brief psychotic disorder. This disorder is characterized by psychotic symptoms, such as the delusion that someone is trying to harm her. The symptoms last up to one month and commonly occur following a stressful life event (e.g., failing an important examination).

12

Mood Disorders

I. DEFINITION, CATEGORIES, AND EPIDEMIOLOGY

Patient snapshot 12-1. A 35-year-old man comes to his physician complaining of tiredness and mild headaches, which have been present for the past 8 months. The patient relates that he is not interested in playing basketball, a game he formerly enjoyed, nor does he have much interest in sex. The patient denies that he is depressed but tells the physician, "Maybe I am more trouble to my family than I am worth." Physical examination is unremarkable except that the patient has lost 10 pounds since his last visit 1 year ago.

What is wrong with this patient? (see III A 1 and Table 12-1)

A. **Definition.** In mood disorders, emotions that the individual cannot control cause **serious distress** and **occupational problems, social problems,** or both.

B. The **major categories** are:

1. **Major depressive disorder.** Patients with this disorder have recurrent episodes of depression (i.e., loss of pleasure and interest in usual activities, hopelessness, suicidality), each episode lasting at least 2 weeks.

2. **Bipolar disorder**
   a. **Bipolar I disorder.** Patients have episodes of both mania (i.e., elevated mood) and depression.
   b. **Bipolar II disorder.** Patients have episodes of both hypomania (i.e., elevated mood that is not as severe as in mania) and depression.

3. **Dysthymic disorder.** Patients with this disorder are mildly depressed (dysthymia) most of the time for at least 2 years, with no discrete episodes of illness.

4. **Cyclothymic disorder.** Patients have dysthymia and hypomania lasting at least two years with no discreet episodes. Many affected patients have relatives with bipolar disorder.

C. Epidemiology

1. **Lifetime prevalence**
   a. The lifetime prevalence of major depressive disorder is about **two times higher in women than in men.**
   b. The lifetime prevalence of **bipolar disorder is about equal for both sexes.**

2. **No ethnic differences** are found in the occurrence of mood disorders. Because of limited access to health care, bipolar disorder in poor African-American and

Table 12-1
Symptoms of Depression and Mania

Symptom	Likelihood of Occurrence
Depression	
Feelings of sadness, hopelessness, helplessness, and low self-esteem	+++
Reduced interest or pleasure in most activities	+++
Reduced energy and motivation	+++
Feelings of anxiety and guilt	+++
Sleep problems (e.g,. waking frequently at night and too early in the morning)	+++
Difficulty with memory and concentration	++
Physically slowed down (particularly in the elderly) or agitated	++
Decreased appetite for food and decreased libido	++
Depressive feelings are worse in the morning than in the evening	++
Suicidal thoughts	++
Makes suicide attempt or commits suicide	+
Delusions of destruction and fatal illness	+
Mania	
Strong feelings of mental and physical well-being	+++
Feelings of self-importance	+++
Irritability and impulsivity	+++
Uncharacteristic lack of modesty in dress or behavior	+++
Inability to control aggressive impulses	+++
Inability to concentrate on relevant stimuli	+++
Compelled to speak quickly (pressured speech)	+++
Thoughts move rapidly from one to the other (flight of ideas)	+++
Impaired judgment	+++
False beliefs (delusions), often of power and influence	++

+++ = seen in most patients.
++ = seen in many patients.
+ = seen in some patients.

Hispanic patients may progress to a point at which the condition is misdiagnosed as schizophrenia.

II. ETIOLOGY

A. Biologic factors

1. **Neurotransmitter activity** is altered in patients with mood disorders (see Chapter 9).

2. **Abnormalities of the limbic-hypothalamic-pituitary-adrenal axis** are seen. The **dexamethasone suppression test,** which measures the regulation of cortisol production, is used to diagnose depression (see Chapter 16).

3. **Immune system function** (see Chapter 20) and **sleep patterns** (see Chapter 7) may be abnormal in patients with mood disorders.

B. Psychosocial factors

1. The **loss of a parent in the first decade of life** and the **loss of a spouse** or child in adulthood correlate with major depressive disorder.

2. **"Learned helplessness"** (i.e., when attempts to escape a bad situation prove futile; see Chapter 5), **low self-esteem,** and **loss of hope** may be related to the development of depression.

3. Psychosocial factors are **not involved in the etiology of mania or hypomania.**

III. CLINICAL SIGNS AND SYMPTOMS

A. Depression (Table 12-1)

1. Some patients seem unaware of or deny depression (i.e., **masked depression**), even though symptoms are present.

2. Patients who experience delusions or hallucinations while depressed have **depression with psychotic features.**

3. **Seasonal affective disorder (SAD)** is a subtype of major depressive disorder associated with short day length; treatment involves increasing light exposure using artificial lighting.

4. The symptoms of depression in both major depressive disorder and bipolar disorder are **similar.**

B. **Mania** (see Table 12-1). In contrast to depressed patients, manic patients are quickly identified because **judgment is impaired,** and the patient may violate the law.

IV. DIFFERENTIAL DIAGNOSIS, PROGNOSIS, AND TREATMENT

A. **Differential diagnosis.** Certain medical diseases, neurologic disorders, and psychiatric disorders and use of prescription drugs are associated with mood symptoms (Table 12-2).

B. Prognosis

1. **Depression is a self-limiting disorder,** with each **episode lasting 6–12 months.**

2. A **manic episode is also self-limiting, each lasts approximately 3 months.**

3. Patients with major depressive disorder and bipolar disorder usually are **mentally healthy between episodes.**

C. Treatment. Depression is successfully treated in most patients. However, **because of the social stigma associated with mental illness,** only approximately 25% of patients with major depression seek and receive treatment.

Table 12-2
Other Causes of Mood Symptoms

Category	Cause
Medical	Pancreatic and other cancers; renal and cardiopulmonary disease
Endocrine	Thyroid, adrenal, or parathyroid dysfunction
Infectious	Pneumonia, mononucleosis, AIDS
Inflammatory	Systemic lupus erythematosus, rheumatoid arthritis
Neurologic	Parkinson disease, epilepsy, multiple sclerosis, stroke, brain trauma or tumor, dementia
Nutritional	Nutritional deficiency
Prescription drugs	Reserpine, propranolol, steroids, methyldopa, oral contraceptives
Psychiatric disorder	Drug and alcohol abuse and withdrawal, anxiety disorders, schizophrenia, eating disorders, somatization disorder

AIDS = acquired immune deficiency syndrome.

1. **Pharmacologic treatment**
   a. The effects of antidepressant agents are usually seen in **3–6 weeks.**
   b. **Selective serotonin reuptake inhibitors (SSRIs) are often used** as first-line agents, because they have limited adverse effects (see Chapter 10).
   c. **Lithium** is the drug of choice for patients with **bipolar disorder.** Anticonvulsants are also effective (see Chapter 10).

2. Under specific circumstances (see Chapter 10), **electroconvulsive therapy (ECT)** is used to treat mood disorders.

3. **Psychological treatment**
   a. Psychological treatment of mood disorders includes interpersonal, family, behavioral, cognitive, and psychoanalytic therapy.
   b. **Psychological treatment in conjunction with pharmacologic treatment** is more effective than either form of treatment alone for depression and dysthymia.
   c. **Pharmacologic treatment** is most effective for bipolar disorder and cyclothymic disorder.

Answer to Patient Snapshot Question

12-1. This patient is suffering from "masked" depression. He denies that he is depressed, even though symptoms of depression (e.g., vague physical complaints, lack of interest in former activities, lack of interest in sex, and weight loss) have been present for the past 8 months.

13

Cognitive Disorders

I. OVERVIEW

A. Etiology

    1. Cognitive disorders (formerly called organic mental syndromes) are caused primarily by abnormalities in the chemistry, structure, or physiology of the brain.

    2. The problem may originate in the brain or may result from physical illness.

B. Types. The major cognitive disorders are **delirium, dementia, and amnestic disorder.** Characteristics of these disorders are listed in Table 13-1.

C. Major features

    1. The hallmarks of cognitive disorders are **cognitive problems,** such as **deficits in memory, orientation, or judgment.**

    2. Mood changes, anxiety, irritability, paranoia, and psychosis, if present, are secondary to the cognitive loss.

II. DEMENTIA OF THE ALZHEIMER TYPE (ALZHEIMER DISEASE)

A. Diagnosis

    1. Alzheimer dementia is the **most common type of dementia.** In confused elderly persons depression must first be ruled out, because depressed patients also have cognitive problems (Chapter 12).

    2. Normal aging is associated with reduced ability to learn new information quickly and a general slowing of mental processes. In contrast to Alzheimer disease, changes associated with normal aging do not interfere with normal activities.

B. Clinical course

    1. Patients show a **gradual loss of memory and intellectual abilities,** inability to control impulses, and lack of judgment.

    2. Later in the illness, symptoms include confusion and psychosis that progress to coma and **death** (usually **8 to 10 years from diagnosis**).

C. Pathophysiology

    1. A number of gross and microscopic **neuroanatomic, neurophysiologic, neurotransmitter and genetic factors** are implicated in Alzheimer disease (Table 13-2).

    2. Alzheimer disease is **seen more commonly in women;** estrogen replacement therapy may have a protective effect in postmenopausal women.

Table 13-1
Characteristics of the Cognitive Disorders

Characteristic	Delirium	Dementia	Amnestic Disorder
PATIENT SNAPSHOT	Three days after surgery to repair an aortic aneurysm, a 70-year-old woman with no psychiatric history seems confused and frightened.	A 76-year-old retired banker is alert but cannot relate what day, month, or year it is, nor can he identify the object in his hand as a cup.	An alert 50-year-old man with a 30-year history of alcoholism claims that he was born in 1985.
Hallmark	Impaired consciousness	Loss of memory and intellectual abilities, but with a normal level of consciousness	Loss of memory, with few other cognitive problems and a normal level of consciousness
Occurrence	• More common in children and the elderly • Causes psychiatric symptoms in medical and surgical patients	• Increased incidence with age • Seen in about 20% of individuals older than age 65	• Patients commonly have a history of alcohol abuse
Etiology	• CNS disease, trauma, or infection • Systemic disease • High fever • Substance abuse • Substance withdrawal	• Alzheimer disease • Vascular disease • CNS disease, trauma, or infection (e.g., HIV)	• Thiamine deficiency due to long-term alcohol abuse, leading to destruction of mediotemporal lobe structures (Korsakoff syndrome) • Temporal lobe trauma, disease, or infection • Herpes simplex encephalitis
Associated physical findings	• Acute medical illness • Autonomic dysfunction • Abnormal EEG	• No medical illness • Little autonomic dysfunction • Normal EEG	• No medical illness • Little autonomic dysfunction • Normal EEG
Associated psychological findings	• Poor orientation to person, place, and time • Illusions or hallucinations • Anxiety and agitation • Worsening of symptoms at night	• No psychotic symptoms • Depression • Little diurnal variability	• No psychotic symptoms • Depression • Little diurnal variability
Course	• Develops quickly • Fluctuating course with lucid intervals	• Develops slowly • Progressive course	• Course dependent on the cause
Treatment and prognosis	• Reduce external sensory stimuli • Identify and treat the underlying medical cause and symptoms usually remit	• Provide medical and psychological support • Usually irreversible	• Identify and treat the underlying medical cause • May be temporary or chronic, depending on the cause

CNS = central nervous system; EEG = electroencephalogram.

Table 13-2

Pathophysiology of Alzheimer Disease

Category	Characteristics
Gross neuroanatomy	• Enlarged ventricles, diffuse atrophy, flattened sulci
Microscopic neuroanatomy	• Senile plaques and neurofibrillary tangles (also seen in Down syndrome and, to a lesser extent, in normal aging) • Loss of cholinergic neurons in the basal forebrain • Neuronal loss and degeneration in the hippocampus and cortex
Neurophysiology	• Reduction in brain levels of choline acetyltransferase, which is needed to synthesize acetylcholine • Abnormal processing of amyloid precursor protein • Decreased membrane fluidity as a result of abnormal regulation of membrane phospholipid metabolism
Neurotransmitters	• Hypoactivity of acetylcholine and norepinephrine • Abnormal activity of somatostatin, vasoactive intestinal polypeptide, and corticotropin
Genetic associations	• Abnormalities of chromosome 21 (as in Down syndrome) • Abnormalities of chromosomes 1 and 14 (implicated particularly in Alzheimer occurring before age 65 years) • Possession of at least one copy of the apo E_4 gene on chromosome 19

D. Treatment

    1. **Pharmacologic interventions** include:

        a. **Psychotropic agents** to treat associated symptoms of anxiety, depression, or psychosis

        b. **Acetylcholinesterase inhibitors.** Tacrine (Cognex), donepezil (Aricept), rivastigmine (Exelon), and galantamine (Reminyl), a new agent, are used to temporarily **slow progression** of the disease. These agents cannot restore function already lost.

    2. The most effective **behavioral interventions** involve providing a structured environment, including:

        a. Putting labels on doors identifying the room's function

        b. Providing daily written information about time, date, and year

        c. Providing daily written activity schedules

        d. Providing practical safety measures (e.g., disconnecting the stove)

14

Other Psychiatric Disorders

I. ANXIETY DISORDERS

Patient snapshot 14-1. A 40-year-old man tells his physician that he is frequently troubled, particularly during the night, by thoughts that he will die in an accident. The patient says that whenever he starts to worry about this, he feels better if he gets out of bed to make sure that the stove is turned off. He reports that he is often tired because he gets up so frequently during the night.

What disorder is this man suffering from, and what is the most effective treatment? (see Table 14-1 and I C 2)

A. Characteristics

   1. **Fear** is a normal reaction to a known environmental source of danger. Individuals with **anxiety** experience apprehension, but the **source of danger is unknown or is inadequate to account for the symptoms.**

   2. The **physical characteristics** of anxiety are similar to those of fear. They include restlessness, shakiness, dizziness, palpitations (subjective experience of tachycardia), mydriasis (pupil dilation), tingling in the extremities, numbness around the mouth, gastrointestinal disturbances such as diarrhea, and urinary frequency.

   3. **Organic causes** of anxiety include excessive caffeine intake, substance abuse, vitamin B_{12} deficiency, hyperthyroidism, hypoglycemia, anemia, pulmonary disease, cardiac arrhythmia, and pheochromocytoma (adrenal tumor).

   4. The **neurotransmitters** involved in the manifestations of anxiety include decreased gamma-aminobutyric acid (GABA) and serotonin activity, and increased norepinephrine activity (see Chapter 9).

B. **Classification.** The *Diagnostic and Statistical Manual of Mental Disorders*, 4th edition (DSM-IV), classification of anxiety disorders includes **panic disorder, phobias, obsessive-compulsive disorder, posttraumatic stress disorder, and generalized anxiety disorder.** Adjustment disorder often must be distinguished from posttraumatic stress disorder (Table 14-1).

C. Treatment

   1. **Benzodiazepines and buspirone** are used to treat anxiety (see Chapter 10). The **β-blockers** are used also, particularly to control the **autonomic symptoms of anxiety.**

   2. **Antidepressants,** particularly the selective serotonin reuptake inhibitors (**SSRIs**) [see Chapter 10], are the most effective long-term therapy for **panic disorder and obsessive-compulsive disorder.**

Table 14-1
DSM-IV Classification of the Anxiety Disorders and Adjustment Disorder

Classification	Characteristics
Panic disorder*	• Episodic (about twice weekly) periods of intense anxiety with a sudden onset, each episode lasting approximately 30 minutes • Cardiac and respiratory symptoms and feelings of impending doom • More common in young women in their 20s • Attacks can be induced by administration of sodium lactate or CO_2 • Strong genetic component
Phobias (specific and social)	• Irrational fear of specific things (e.g., snakes, airplane travel) or social situations (e.g., public speaking, eating in public, using public restrooms) • Because of the fear, the patient avoids the object or social situation; this avoidance leads to social and occupational problems
Obsessive-compulsive disorder	• Recurrent unwanted, intrusive thoughts, feelings, and images (i.e., obsessions), which cause anxiety • Performing repetitive actions (i.e., compulsions, such as hand washing) relieves the anxiety • Patients have insight (i.e., they realize that the obsessions and compulsions are irrational and want to eliminate them)
Generalized anxiety disorder	• Persistent anxiety symptoms lasting 6 months or more • Gastrointestinal symptoms are common • Symptoms are not related to a specific person or situation (i.e., symptoms are "free-floating")
Posttraumatic stress disorder (PTSD) and acute stress disorder (ASD)	• Emotional symptoms, intrusive memories, guilt, and dissociative symptoms occurring after a potentially catastrophic or life-threatening event (e.g., rape earthquake, fire, serious accident) • In PTSD, symptoms last for > 1 month and can last for years • In ASD, symptoms last only between 2 days and 4 weeks
Adjustment disorder	• Emotional symptoms (e.g., anxiety, depression, conduct problems) causing social, school, or work impairment that occur within 3 months and lasts less than 6 months after a stressful life event (e.g., divorce, bankruptcy, moving)

DSM-IV = *Diagnostic and Statistical Manual of Mental Disorders,* 4th edition.
*Panic disorder may or may not be associated with agoraphobia (i.e., fear of open places, or situations involving the inability to escape or to obtain help).

II. SOMATOFORM DISORDERS, FACTITIOUS DISORDER, AND MALINGERING

Patient snapshot 14-2. A 50-year-old man reports that he has felt "sick" and "weak" for the last 10 years. He frequently changes physicians when they cannot find anything wrong with him. He often misses work because he feels ill, and he now fears that he has cancer. Physical examination is unremarkable.

What diagnosis best fits this clinical picture, and what is the most effective treatment? (see Table 14-2 and II A 4)

A. Characteristics, classification, and treatment

    1. Patients with somatoform disorders are characterized as having **physical symptoms without sufficient organic cause.** The most important **differential diagnosis** is **unidentified organic disease.**

Table 14-2
DSM-IV Classification of Somatoform Disorders

Classification	Characteristics
Somatization disorder	• History of multiple physical complaints (e.g., nausea, dyspnea, menstrual problems) over years • Onset before 30 years of age
Conversion disorder	• Sudden loss of sensory or motor function (e.g., blindness, paralysis) • Often associated with a stressful life event • Patients appear relatively unconcerned (*la belle indifference*) • More common in adolescents and young adults
Hypochondriasis	• Exaggerated concern with health and illness lasting > 6 months • Patient goes to different physicians seeking help ("doctor shopping") • More common in middle and old age
Body dysmorphic disorder	• Normal-appearing patients believe they appear abnormal • Patients may refuse to appear in public • Onset usually in the late teens
Pain disorder	• Intense, prolonged pain not explained completely by physical disease • Onset usually in the 30s and 40s

DSM-IV = *Diagnostic and Statistical Manual of Mental Disorders,* 4th edition.

   2. The DSM-IV categories of somatoform disorders and their characteristics are listed in Table 14-2.

   3. With the exception of hypochondriasis, which is seen equally in men and women, the somatoform disorders are more common in women.

   4. Treatment includes forming a good physician-patient relationship, including scheduling regular appointments and providing ongoing reassurance.

 B. Factitious disorder and malingering. Individuals with somatoform disorders truly believe that they are ill, but patients with factitious and related disorders **feign illness for psychological or tangible gain** (Table 14-3).

III. PERSONALITY DISORDERS

   Patient snapshot 14-3. A 40-year-old man asks his physician to see him first whenever he has an appointment with her. The patient states that the physician should not be annoyed by this request, but instead should understand that he is "superior" to her other patients.

What personality disorder best fits this clinical picture? (see Table 14-4)

 A. Characteristics and classification

   1. Patients with personality disorders have **long-standing, rigid, unsuitable patterns of relating to others** that cause social and occupational problems.

   2. Personality disorders are categorized by the DSM-IV into **three clusters—clusters A, B, and C—**each with specific characteristics and familial associations (Table 14-4).

 B. Treatment. Patients with personality disorders usually are not aware of their problems and do not seek psychiatric help. Individual and group psychotherapy may be useful for those who seek help.

Table 14-3
DSM-IV Classification of Factitious Disorder and Malingering

Classification	Characteristics
Factitious disorder*	• Conscious simulation or induction of physical or psychiatric illness for the purpose of receiving attention from medical personnel • Patient undergoes unnecessary medical and surgical procedures • May have a "grid abdomen" (multiple crossed scars from repeated surgeries)
Factitious disorder by proxy	• Conscious simulation or induction of physical or psychiatric illness in another person, typically in a child by a parent, to receive attention from medical personnel • Is a form of child abuse and must be reported to child welfare authorities
Malingering	• Conscious simulation of physical or psychiatric illness for financial or other obvious gain • Avoids treatment by medical personnel • Health complaints cease when the desired gain is achieved

DSM-IV = *Diagnostic and Statistical Manual of Mental Disorders,* 4th edition.
*Formerly called Munchausen syndrome

IV. DISSOCIATIVE DISORDERS

 Patient snapshot 14-4. A 30-year-old salesman from New Jersey is found working in a strip mall in Ohio. He does not remember his former life nor how he got to Ohio. His level of consciousness is normal, and there is no evidence of head injury.

What diagnosis best fits this clinical picture? (see Table 14-5)

A. Characteristics

  1. The dissociative disorders are characterized by **temporary loss of memory or personal identity or by feelings of detachment** due to psychological factors. There is no psychosis.

  2. These disorders are often related to **disturbing psychological events** in the recent or remote past.

  3. The differential diagnosis of dissociative disorders includes memory loss occurring as a result of **head injury,** substance abuse, or other factors.

B. Classification and treatment

  1. The DSM-IV categories of dissociative disorders are listed in Table 14-5.

  2. Treatment includes **hypnosis, sodium amobarbital interviews** (see Chapter 16), **and psychotherapy** to recover "lost" (repressed) memories.

V. OBESITY AND EATING DISORDERS

 Patient snapshot 14-5. The mother of a 15-year-old girl tells you that she is concerned because she often finds candy and cookie wrappers stuffed under the mattress in her daughter's bedroom. Her daughter is on both the swim team and track team at school and is of normal weight. When questioned, the mother remembers that her daughter had 10 cavities on a recent dental visit.

What is the best diagnosis for this girl and what treatment would be most helpful? (see Table 14-6 and V B 3).

Table 14-4
DSM-IV Classification of Personality Disorders

Classification	Characteristics
Cluster A	**Hallmarks: peculiar, avoids social relationships; not psychotic** **Genetic associations: psychotic illnesses**
Paranoid	• Suspicious, mistrustful, litigious • Responsibility for own problems attributed to others • Doubts the physician's motives when ill
Schizoid	• Lifelong pattern of voluntary social withdrawal without psychosis • Becomes even more withdrawn when ill
Schizotypal	• Peculiar appearance • Odd thought patterns and behavior without psychosis
Cluster B	**Hallmarks: dramatic, erratic** **Genetic associations: mood disorders, substance abuse**
Histrionic	• Extroverted, emotional, sexually provocative behavior • Inability to maintain intimate relationships • Presents symptoms in a dramatic manner when ill
Narcissistic	• Grandiosity, envy, and sense of entitlement • Lack of empathy for others • Illness can threaten self-image • Insists on special treatment when ill
Antisocial	• Inability to conform to social norms; criminality • Diagnosed as conduct disorder in those younger than age 18 • Lay terms are *psychopaths* and *sociopaths*
Borderline	• Unstable; impulsive mood and behavior • Feels bored, empty, and alone • Suicide attempts for trivial reasons • Self-mutilation
Cluster C	**Hallmarks: fearful, anxious** **Genetic association: anxiety disorders**
Avoidant	• Sensitive to rejection • Socially withdrawn and shy • Feels inferior to others
Obsessive-compulsive	• Orderly, stubborn, indecisive • Perfectionistic • Fears loss of control and tries to control the physician when ill
Dependent	• Lack of self-confidence • Lets others assume responsibility • Increased need for the physician's attention when ill
Passive-aggressive*	• Procrastination, stubbornness, and inefficiency • Seeming compliance, but actual defiance • Fails to comply with treatment recommendations

DSM-IV = *Diagnostic and Statistical Manual of Mental Disorders,* 4th edition.
*Passive-aggressive personality disorder is no longer a DSM diagnosis; description of it is now in the DSM-IV Appendix.

Table 14-5
DSM-IV Classification of Dissociative Disorders

Classification	Characteristics
Dissociative amnesia	• Inability to remember important personal information
Dissociative fugue	• Amnesia combined with sudden wandering from home and taking on a different identity
Dissociative identity disorder (formerly called multiple personality disorder)	• At least two separate personalities within an individual • More common in women • Associated with sexual abuse in childhood
Depersonalization disorder	• Persistent, recurrent feelings of detachment from one's own body, a social situation, or the environment (derealization)

DSM-IV = *Diagnostic and Statistical Manual of Mental Disorders,* 4th edition.

Table 14-6
Obesity and Eating Disorders

Classification	Psychological/social characteristics	Physiological characteristics
Obesity	• Occurs in more than 25% of adults in the United States • Strong genetic factors • More common in lower socioeconomic groups	• Body weight at least 20% more than ideal (per standard charts) • Increased risk for cardiovascular disease, some cancers, osteoarthritis, diabetes mellitus, respiratory problems
Anorexia nervosa	• Excessive dieting • Abnormal eating habits (e.g., simulating eating) • Disturbance of body image; overwhelming fear of becoming obese • Lack of interest in sex • Excessive exercising • Abuse of laxatives, diuretics, and/or enemas • Most common in adolescents and young adults • High academic achievement • Interfamily conflicts particularly between mother and daughter • Normal mood	• Severe weight loss (losing $\geq$ 15% body weight) • Normal appetite but refusal to eat • Amenorrhea (three or more missed menstrual periods) • Lanugo (downy body hair on trunk) • Melanosis coli (blackened area on the colon if there is laxative abuse) • Increased risk for osteoporosis • Mild anemia and leukopenia • Electrolyte disturbances
Bulimia nervosa	• Secretive binge eating followed by induced vomiting • Excessive exercising • Abuse of laxatives, diuretics, and/or enemas • Poor self image • Depression	• Normal body weight • Esophageal varices caused by repeated vomiting • Erosion of tooth enamel due to gastric acid in the mouth • Swelling or infection of the parotid glands • Callouses on the dorsal surface of the hand from inducing gagging • Electrolyte disturbances

A. **Classification and characteristics**

1. **Obesity and the eating disorders anorexia nervosa and bulimia nervosa occur more often in women** than in men (Table 14-6).

2. Anorexia and bulimia are more common during teenage years and in higher socioeconomic groups.

B. **Treatment**

1. **Treatment for obesity.** Commercial dieting and weight loss programs and surgical techniques are initially effective in the treatment of obesity, but are of little value in maintaining long-term weight loss. Most often, all lost weight is regained within 5 years. The most effective long-term treatment is a combination of diet and exercise.

2. **Treatment for anorexia nervosa.** This life-threatening condition is treated initially by hospitalization to restore nutritional status. Family therapy is the most useful form of psychotherapy for this disorder.

3. **Treatment for bulimia nervosa** includes psychotherapy or behavioral therapy.

4. Antidepressants, particularly the SSRIs, are more useful for bulimia nervosa than for anorexia nervosa.

VI. NEUROPSYCHIATRIC DISORDERS IN CHILDHOOD

A. **Classification.** These childhood disorders include **pervasive developmental disorders, attention deficit hyperactivity disorder (ADHD), disruptive behavior disorders, Tourette syndrome, separation anxiety disorder, and selective mutism.** Their characteristics are shown in Table 14-7.

B. **Incidence.** With the exception of Rett disorder and selective mutism, all of these disorders are **more common in boys** than in girls.

Answers to Patient Snapshot Questions

14-1. This man is suffering from obsessive compulsive disorder (OCD), which is an anxiety disorder. He is troubled by recurrent, unwanted thoughts (obsessions) about violent death; these obsessions are relieved by engaging in repetitive actions (checking the stove). The most effective long-term treatment for OCD is antidepressant medication, particularly the selective serotonin reuptake inhibitors.

14-2. This patient is suffering from hypochondriasis, a somatoform disorder. He is not physically ill but has exaggerated concerns about illness and goes "doctor shopping" to get help. The most effective treatment is for the physician to provide support, schedule regular appointments, and give reassurance to this patient.

14-3. The disorder that best fits this clinical picture is narcissistic personality disorder. People with this disorder have a sense of special entitlement and often insist on special treatment by others, including physicians.

14-4. This man is probably suffering from dissociative fugue. People with this psychological disorder have a normal level of consciousness, but have memory problems coupled with wandering away from home.

14-5. This 15-year-old girl is probably suffering from bulimia nervosa, which involves binge eating and then purging to avoid weight gain. Evidence for secretive ingestion of high calorie foods and dental caries due to erosion of tooth enamel from vomiting provide evidence of this condition. Treatment for bulimia includes psychotherapy and antidepressant medication.

Table 14-7
Neuropsychiatric Disorders in Childhood

Classification	Characteristics
Pervasive Developmental Disorders	
Autistic disorder	• Begins before age 3 years; is rare • Severe communication problems despite normal hearing • Significant problems forming social relationships, including those with caregivers • Repetitive behavior (e.g., spinning, self-injury) • Unusual abilities (e.g., calculating) in some children, known as *savants* • Intelligence is usually subnormal • Neurological (not psychological) etiology • History of perinatal complications • Genetic component • Treatment involves increasing social, communication, and self-care skills • Poor prognosis; few can live and work independently
Asperger disorder	• A mild form of autistic disorder • Significant problems forming social relationships • Repetitive behavior • Normal verbal and cognitive skills
Rett disorder	• Loss of social, verbal, and cognitive development leading to mental retardation after up to 4 years of normal functioning • Seen only in girls; is X-linked and affected males die before birth • Stereotyped hand-wringing movements
ADHD and Disruptive Behavior Disorders	
ADHD	• Begins in early childhood • Is relatively common, occurring in 3% to 5% of children • Hyperactivity and/or limited attention span • Prone to accidents • Impulsivity, emotional lability, irritability • Minor brain dysfunction • Normal intelligence • Treated with CNS stimulants, such as methylphenidate [Ritalin, Concerta (a long-acting form)] or pemoline (Cylert); may also be treated with antidepressants (e.g., imipramine) • In 20% of patients, the characteristics persist into adulthood
Conduct disorder	• Persistent behavior that violates social norms (e.g. harming animals, stealing, fire-setting) • At age 18 and older, this disorder is diagnosed as antisocial personality disorder (see Table 14-4)
Oppositional defiant disorder	• Persistent defiant, negative, and noncompliant behavior (e.g., argumentativeness, resentment) toward authority figures (e.g., parents, teachers) • Does not grossly violate social norms
Other Disorders of Childhood	
Tourette disorder	• Onset before age 18 years and usually at 7 to 8 years of age; is rare • Motor and vocal tics • Involuntary use of profanity • Genetic relationship to ADHD and obsessive-compulsive disorder • Haloperidol is the primary treatment; pimozide is also effective • Lifelong chronic symptoms

(continued)

Table 14-7—*Continued*

Neuropsychiatric Disorders in Childhood

Classification	Characteristics
Separation anxiety disorder	• Overwhelming fear of the loss of a major attachment figure (e.g., mother) • Production of physical complaints to avoid going to school • Most common onset age is 7 to 8 years; may occur in preschool years
Selective mutism	• Refusal to speak in some or all social situations; child may communicate with gestures • Not normal shyness • More common in girls

ADHD = attention deficit hyperactivity disorder; CNS = central nervous system.

15

Suicide

 Patient snapshot 15-1. A hospitalized, depressed 18-year-old girl tells her physician that she plans to kill herself with her father's gun when she is released from the hospital. She insists on going home. The father wants his daughter to come home and promises to get rid of the gun.

What should the physician do? (see II B)

I. EPIDEMIOLOGY

A. Suicide is the **ninth leading cause of death** in the United States, after heart disease, cancer, stroke, chronic obstructive pulmonary disease, accidents, pneumonia, diabetes mellitus, and AIDS.

B. The **suicide rate** in the United States is in the midrange of that of other developed countries.

II. SUICIDAL BEHAVIOR

A. Attempts

1. There are approximately **nine times more suicide attempts** than actual suicides. Approximately 30% of people who attempt suicide try again, and 10% succeed.

2. Although women attempt suicide four times more often than men do, **men successfully commit suicide three times more often than women do.**

B. **Clinical assessment.** Clinicians should **assess suicide risk** during every examination of patients who might have a depressed mood.

1. If the threat is serious and the patient is hospitalized, suggest that the patient remain in the hospital.

2. **Emergency or involuntary hospitalization** is used for patients who cannot or will not agree to hospitalization and requires the certification of one or two physicians. Depending on individual state law, the patient can be held for 15 to 60 days before a court hearing.

III. RISK FACTORS (Table 15-1)

A. **Hierarchy of risk.** The five highest risk factors for suicide (in decreasing order of risk) are:

1. Serious prior suicide attempt

2. Older than 45 years of age

Table 15-1
Risk Factors for Suicide

Factor	Increased Risk	Decreased Risk
Gender	Male	Female
Age	• Middle aged and elderly • Adolescence (third leading cause of death in this group)	• Children • Young adult (age 25 to 40 years)
Occupation	• Professional	• Nonprofessional
Ethnicity and religion	• Caucasian • Jewish • Protestant	• Non-Caucasian • Catholic • Muslim
Social and work relationships	• Unmarried, divorced, or widowed (particularly men) • Lives alone • Unemployed	• Married • Strong social support systems • Has children • Employed
Family history	• Parent committed suicide • Early loss of a parent through divorce or death	• No family history of suicide • Intact family in childhood
Psychiatric picture	• Severe depression • Psychotic symptoms • Hopelessness • Impulsiveness	• Mild depression • No psychotic symptoms • Some hopefulness • Thinks things out
Health	• Serious medical illness	• Good health
Previous suicidal behavior	• Serious prior suicide attempt • Rescue was remote • < 3 months since the last attempt	• No prior attempt • Rescue was inevitable • > 3 months since the last attempt
Method	• Self-inflicted gunshot wound • Crashing one's vehicle • Hanging oneself • Jumping from a high place	• Overdose of pills • Slashing one's wrists

3. Alcohol dependence

4. History of rage and violent behavior

5. Male gender

B. Depression

1. **Patients recovering from severe depression are at higher risk** for committing suicide than those who are still severely depressed. The reason for this is that these patients have regained enough clarity of thought and energy to act on their suicidal ideas.

2. The **sudden appearance of peacefulness** in a previously agitated, depressed patient is another risk factor for suicide. This may indicate that the patient has reached an internal decision to kill himself and is now calm.

3. **Depressed patients who believe that they have a serious illness are at increased risk.** Most patients who commit suicide have visited a physician with a physical complaint in the **6 months prior to the act.**

C. Occupation. The risk of suicide is increased among professional women, especially physicians. High-risk professions for both sexes include dentists, police officers, attorneys, and musicians.

D. A plan for suicide. Those who have a plan for and possess an effective means of committing suicide (e.g., drugs and guns) are at increased risk.

Answer to Patient Snapshot Question

15-1. The physician should suggest to the patient that she remain in the hospital. If she refuses, the physician should hold the patient involuntarily until a court hearing can be held to determine if she is a danger to herself. Getting rid of the gun will not eliminate the risk of suicide in this patient.

16

Tests to Determine Psychological and Biological Functioning

 Patient snapshot 16-1. A 51-year-old man presents to his primary care physician on a number of occasions over a period of one year complaining of physical ailments for which no obvious cause can be found. The physician suspects that the patient is depressed (see Chapter 12).

What psychological test can this physician use to augment her diagnostic impressions? (see Table 16-2)

I. PSYCHOLOGICAL TESTS

A. **Types of tests**

    1. Psychological tests are used to assess **intelligence, achievement, personality, and psychopathology.**

    2. These tests are classified by **functional area** assessed and by whether **information is gathered objectively or projectively.**

B. **Objective versus projective tests**

    1. An **objective test** is based on questions that are **easily scored** and statistically analyzed.

    2. A **projective test** requires the subject to **interpret the questions.** Responses are assumed to be based on the subject's motivational state and defense mechanisms.

Table 16-1
IQ and the Classification of Average and Below-Average Intelligence

IQ*	Classification
< 20	Profound mental retardation
20–40	Severe mental retardation
35–55	Moderate mental retardation
50–70	Mild mental retardation
71–89	Borderline to low average intelligence
90–109	Average intelligence

IQ = intelligence quotient; DSM-IV = *Diagnostic and Statistical Manual of Mental Disorders,* 4th edition; WAIS-R = Wechsler Adult Intelligence Scale-Revised.
*Overlaps in IQ scores are due to differences in DSM-IV and WAIS-R scales.

3. The results of any psychological test can be influenced by **culture and early experiences** as well as by the characteristic being measured.

II. INTELLIGENCE TESTS

A. Intelligence and mental age

   1. **Intelligence** is defined as the ability to reason; understand abstract concepts; assimilate facts; recall, analyze, and organize information; and meet the requirements of a new situation.

   2. **Mental age,** as defined by Alfred Binet, is the average intellectual level of people of a specific chronological age.

B. Intelligence quotient (IQ)

   1. On the **Stanford-Binet scale,** IQ is the ratio of mental age (MA) to chronological age (CA) multiplied by 100. That is, IQ = MA/CA × 100.

      a. An **IQ of 100** indicates that the person's mental and chronological ages are the same.

      b. The standard deviation in IQ scores is about 15 points. An individual with an IQ that is more than two standard deviations lower than the mean (IQ < 70) is usually considered **mentally retarded** (Table 16-1).

      c. IQ is relatively **stable throughout life.** An individual's IQ is usually the same in old age as in childhood. The highest chronological age used to determine IQ is about 15 years.

   2. Biological factors associated with IQ

      a. IQ has a **strong genetic component.** IQ is concordant in about 85% of monozygotic twins reared together and 67% of monozygotic twins reared apart.

      b. Although primarily genetic, **poor nutrition and illness** during development can negatively affect IQ.

C. Wechsler intelligence tests

   1. The **Wechsler Adult Intelligence Scale-Revised (WAIS-R)** is the most commonly used intelligence test.

   2. The WAIS-R has **11 subtests, 6 verbal and 5 performance.** The subtests evaluate general information, comprehension, similarities, arithmetic, vocabulary, picture assembly, picture completion, block design, object assembly, digit span, and digit symbol.

   3. The **Wechsler Intelligence Scale for Children-Revised (WISC-R)** is used to test children 6 to 16½ years of age.

   4. The **Wechsler Preschool and Primary Scale of Intelligence (WPPSI)** is used to test children 4 to 6½ years of age.

III. ACHIEVEMENT TESTS

A. Uses

   1. Achievement tests evaluate how well an individual has mastered **specific instructional content.**

   2. These tests are used for evaluation and career counseling in schools and industry.

B. Specific achievement tests

   1. The **Wide-Range Achievement Test (WRAT),** which is frequently used in medicine, evaluates arithmetic, reading, and spelling skills.

    2. **Other achievement tests** include the California, Iowa, Peabody, and Stanford Achievement Tests, as well as the Medical College Admissions Test (MCAT) and the United States Medical Licensing Examination (USMLE).

IV. PERSONALITY TESTS

A. Uses

    1. Personality tests are used to evaluate psychopathology (i.e., depression, thought disorders, hypochondriasis) and personality characteristics.

    2. Personality tests are also used to identify defense mechanisms as well as unconscious emotions and conflicts.

B. **Common personality tests** are listed in Table 16-2.

V. NEUROPSYCHOLOGICAL TESTS

A. **Uses.** Neuropsychological tests assess general intelligence, memory, reasoning, orientation, perceptuomotor performance, language function, attention, and concentration in patients with neurologic problems such as dementia and brain damage.

B. Specific tests

    1. The **Halstead-Reitan Battery (HRB)** is used to detect and localize brain lesions and determine their effects.

Table 16-2

Personality Tests

Test	Characteristics	Examples
Minnesota Multiphasic Personality Inventory (MMPI-2)	Patient takes a paper-and-pencil test containing 566 true-or-false questions Useful for primary care physicians, because no training is required for administration or interpretation	"I often feel jealous." "I avoid social situations."
Rorschach Test	Patient gives his interpretation of 10 bilaterally symmetrical ink blot designs (e.g., "Describe what you see in this picture.")	
Thematic Apperception Test (TAT)	Patient creates a verbal scenario based on drawings depicting ambiguous situations (e.g., "Using this picture, make up a story that has a beginning, a middle, and an end.")	
Sentence Completion Test (SCT)	Patient completes short sentences started by the examiner	"I wish . . . " "My father . . . " "Most people . . . "

(Original source of Rorschach illustration: Kleinmuntz B: *Essentials of Abnormal Psychology.* New York, Harper & Row, 1974. Original source of TAT illustration: Phares EJ: *Clinical Psychology: Concepts, Methods, and Profession,* 2nd edition. Homewood, IL , Dorsey, 1984. Both from Krebs D and Blackman R: *Psychology; A First Encounter.* Harcourt, Brace, Jovanovich, 1988, p. 632. Used by permission of the publisher.)

2. The **Luria-Nebraska Neuropsychological Battery (LNNB)** is used to determine left or right cerebral dominance and to identify specific types of brain dysfunction, such as dyslexia.

3. The **Bender Visual Motor Gestalt Test** is used to evaluate visual and motor ability by recall and reproduction of designs.

VI. PSYCHOLOGICAL EVALUATION OF THE PATIENT WITH PSYCHIATRIC SYMPTOMS

A. Psychiatric history. The patient's psychiatric history is taken as part of the medical history. The psychiatric history includes questions about **mental illness, drug and alcohol use, sexual activity, current living situation, and sources of stress.**

B. Mental status examination

1. The mental status examination evaluates an individual's **current state of mental functioning** (Table 16-3).

2. Terms used to describe psychophysiologic symptoms and mood in patients with psychiatric illness are listed in Table 16-4.

VII. BIOLOGICAL EVALUATION OF THE PATIENT WITH PSYCHIATRIC SYMPTOMS

A. Dexamethasone suppression test (DST)

1. Dexamethasone is a synthetic glucocorticoid. When given to an otherwise healthy individual with a normal hypothalamic-adrenal-pituitary axis, it **suppresses the secretion of cortisol.** In approximately 50% of patients with major depressive disorder, this suppression is limited or absent.

2. Patients with a positive DST result (i.e., those with reduced suppression of cortisol) may **respond well to treatment with antidepressant agents or electroconvulsive therapy.**

3. Positive DST results are not specific. Positive DST results are also seen in **dementia,**

Table 16-3
Variables Evaluated on the Mental Status Examination

Category	Examples
Appearance	Dress, grooming, appearance for age
Attitude toward interviewer	Interested, seductive, defensive, cooperative
Behavior	Posture, gait, eye contact, restlessness
Cognitive functioning	Level of consciousness, memory, orientation
Emotions	Mood, affect
Intellectual functions	Intelligence, judgment, insight
Perception	Depersonalization, illusions, hallucinations
Speech	Rate, clarity, vocabulary abnormalities, volume
Thought process and content	Loose associations, delusions, ideas of reference

Table 16-4
Psychophysiologic States

Mood
Euphoria: strong feelings of elation
Expansive mood: feelings of self-importance and generosity
Euthymic mood: normal mood, with no significant depression or elevation of mood
Dysphoric mood: subjectively unpleasant feeling
Anhedonia: inability to feel pleasure

Affect
Restricted affect: decreased display of emotional responses
Blunted affect: strongly decreased display of emotional responses
Flat affect: complete lack of emotional responses
Labile affect: sudden alterations in emotional responses not related to environmental events

Consciousness and Attention
Normal: alert, can follow commands, normal verbal responses (Glasgow Coma Scale score of 15)
Clouding of consciousness: inability to respond normally to external events
Somnolence: abnormal sleepiness
Stupor: little or no response to environmental stimuli
Coma: total unconsciousness (Glasgow Coma Scale score of 3)

schizophrenia, pregnancy, anorexia nervosa, severe weight loss, endocrine disorders, and the use, abuse, and withdrawal of alcohol and antianxiety agents.

B. Tests of endocrine function

    1. Thyroid function tests are used to evaluate patients for **hypothyroidism** (which mimics **depression**) and **hyperthyroidism** (which mimics **anxiety**).

    2. Patients with depression may have abnormalities in growth hormone, melatonin, gonadotropin, and thyrotropin.

    3. Psychiatric symptoms are seen in endocrine disorders such as **Addison disease and Cushing syndrome.**

C. Measurement of biogenic amines and psychotropic drugs

    1. Abnormalities in both catecholamine and catecholamine metabolite levels are found in some psychiatric syndromes (see Table 9-3).

    2. In some patients, plasma levels of psychotropic drugs are measured to evaluate **compliance,** especially with antipsychotic agents, or to determine whether **therapeutic blood levels** of a drug have been reached, especially with antidepressant agents.

    3. Other tests that are used for psychiatric evaluation are shown in Table 16-5.

Answer to Patient Snapshot Question

16-1. Because no special training is required for administration or interpretation, this primary care physician can use the Minnesota Multiphasic Personality Inventory (MMPI) to augment her psychological assessment of this patient.

Table 16-5
Tests Used in Clinical Psychiatry

Test	Conditions Identified	Description
Electroencephalogram (EEG)	• Epilepsy • Delirium (EEG is usually normal in dementia) • Demyelinating illness	Measures electrical activity in the cortex
Evoked potentials	• Vision and hearing loss in infants • Brain responses in coma	Measures electrical activity in the cortex in response to sensory stimulation
Sodium amobarbital (Amytal) interview	• Conversion disorder • Dissociative disorders	Relaxes patients so that they can express themselves during an interview
Galvanic skin response	• Stress	Measures sweat gland activity; high levels are seen with sympathetic nervous system arousal, resulting in decreased electrical resistance of skin
Sodium lactate administration or CO_2 inhalation	• Panic disorder	Causes panic attacks in susceptible patients
Neuroimaging (CAT, MRI, fMRI, and PET scans)	• Anatomically based brain changes • Demyelinating disease • Metabolism of glucose in neural tissue	Identifies biochemical condition and anatomy of neural tissues and areas of brain activity during specific tasks

CAT = computed axial tomography; MRI = magnetic resonance imaging; fMRI = functional magnetic resonance imaging; PET = positron emission tomography.

17

The Family, Culture, and Illness

I. THE FAMILY

A. Types of families

    1. The traditional **nuclear family** includes a mother, a father, and dependent children living together in **one household.**

    2. The **extended family** includes family members (e.g., grandparents, aunts, and uncles) who live **outside of the household.**

    3. Types of families are listed in Table 17-1.

B. Marriage and children

    1. In the United States, more than **75% of people 30 to 54 years of age are married.**

    2. Married people have **higher self-esteem** and are **mentally and physically healthier** than unmarried people.

    3. In the United States, the cost of raising a child to age 17 is more than $100,000.

C. Divorce

    1. **Close to 50% of all American marriages end in divorce.** Divorced men are more likely than divorced women to remarry.

    2. Factors associated with divorce include short courtship, premarital pregnancy, teenage marriage, divorce in the family, religious or socioeconomic differences, and serious illness or death of a child.

D. Single-parent families

    1. Single-parent families often have **lower incomes and less social support** than two-parent families. As a result, single-parent families are at increased risk for physical and mental illness.

    2. Children in single-parent families are at increased risk for failure in school, depression, drug abuse, suicide, criminal activity, and divorce.

    3. Many unmarried mothers belong to low socioeconomic groups; however, the fastest growing population of single mothers is **educated professional women.**

    4. Types of child custody
        a. In **joint custody,** children spend equal time with both parents.
        b. In **split custody,** each parent has custody of at least one child.
        c. In **sole custody,** children live with one parent and the other has visitation rights.
        d. Fathers are increasingly being granted joint or sole custody.

Table 17-1
Living Arrangements of Children 17 Years Old and Younger in the United States

Type of Family	Approximate Percentage of Children	Comments
Couples with children, one parent employed (usually the father)	23% of all children	The "traditional" family
Couples with children, both parents employed	40% of all children	Increasingly common
Single-parent families, all ethnic groups	28% of all children (62% of African American, 33% of Hispanic, and 21% of white children)	83%–95% are headed by women; 5%–17% are headed by men

E. Family systems theory and family therapy

   1. According to family systems theory, symptoms such as depression or eating disorders are not signs of individual pathology, but indicate **dysfunction** within the family.

   2. Family systems exhibit **homeostasis** (i.e., deviations from typical family patterns occur within a restricted range).

   3. Breakdowns in communication within a **dyad,** or relationship between two family members, result in emotional isolation, and dysfunctional coalitions form between two family members against a third (i.e., a **triangle**).

   4. In family therapy, all members of the family are involved in the treatment of the psychological problem of one family member.

II. UNITED STATES CULTURE

 Patient snapshot 17-1. The principal of a high school is trying to estimate how many of the school's students live in single-parent families.

If the school's population is representative of the United States population, what percent of the students come from single-parent families? (see Table 17-1)

A. **Composition.** The United States has approximately 276 million people, including a variety of **minority subcultures** as well as a **large white middle class** that provides the major cultural influence.

B. Characteristics

   1. **Financial and personal independence** are valued at all ages, especially in the **elderly.**

   2. **Personal hygiene and cleanliness** are emphasized.

   3. The **nuclear family** with few children is valued.

C. **Culture and illness.** Studies show that subcultures respond characteristically to illness (Table 17-2).

D. Culture shock

   1. Culture shock is a strong emotional response to a move to unfamiliar social and

Table 17-2
Characteristics of Ethnic Subcultures in the United States (November, 2000)

Subculture and Approximate Population	Characteristics
African American 35.5 million	• Average income approximately one-half that of white American families • Decreased access to health care services and increased risk of illness and early death (see Table 3-1) • Higher rates of hypertension, heart disease, stroke, obesity, asthma, tuberculosis, diabetes, prostate cancer, and AIDS • Higher death rates from heart disease and most forms of cancer • Lower suicide rate across age groups; equal suicide rate in teenagers • Religion and strong extended kinship networks important in social and personal support
Hispanic American 33 million	• Great value placed on the nuclear family and on large families • Respect for the elderly • Protect elderly relatives from negative medical diagnoses • Make medical decisions for elderly relatives • May seek health care from folk healers (e.g., *chamanes, curanderos espiritistas*) • Religious beliefs play a role in treatment • Emphasis on herbal and botanical remedies • Women are less likely to get mammograms than other ethnic groups • "Hot" and "cold" dietary influences • Dramatic presentation of symptoms
Asian American 11 million	• Children are expected to respect and care for elderly parents • Protect elderly relatives from negative medical diagnoses • Make medical decisions for elderly relatives • Emphasis on education • May express emotional pain as physical illness • Some use folk remedies (e.g., coining, or rubbing a coin on the affected area; resulting bruises are believed to aid the patient) • In some, the abdominal-thoracic area rather than the brain is the spiritual core of the person; the concept of brain death and organ transplant are not well accepted in these groups • Some accumulate acetaldehyde in the metabolism of alcohol, leading to a flushing reaction
Native American 2.5 million	• Receive medical care under the direction of the Indian Health Service of the federal government • The distinction between mental and physical illness is blurred • Engaging in forbidden behavior and witchcraft is thought to cause illness • Incomes are low and rates of alcoholism and suicide are high
White American 227 million	• Anglo-Americans are more stoic and uncomplaining about pain and illness than Americans of Mediterranean descent • May become very ill before seeking treatment • Dramatic style of reporting symptoms • Mediterranean-Americans are more likely to visit physicians and report their medical problems than Anglo-Americans

AIDS = Acquired immune deficiency syndrome.

cultural surroundings. It is reduced by the tendency of immigrants to live in the same geographic area.

2. **Young immigrant men** appear to be at **increased risk for psychiatric problems,** such as paranoid symptoms, schizophrenia, and depression, when compared with other sex and age groups.

Answer to Patient Snapshot Question

17-1. If the school's population is representative of the United States population, 28% if the children live in single-parent families.

18
Sexuality

I. SEXUAL DEVELOPMENT

 Patient snapshot 18-1. While taking a history, a physician learns that a tall, slim 19-year-old woman has never menstruated. External physical examination reveals normal breast development and bilateral inguinal masses. There are no Barr bodies in the buccal smear. A pelvic examination is not performed at this time.

What diagnosis best fits this clinical picture? (see Table 18-1)

A. Prenatal sex determination

    1. Differentiation of the **gonads** is dependent on the presence of the **Y chromosome,** which contains the testis-determining factor gene.

    2. The hormonal secretions of the **testes** direct the differentiation of **male** internal and external genitalia. If testicular hormones are absent during prenatal life, the internal and external genitalia are **female.**

    3. Differential exposure to sex hormones during prenatal life causes **gender differences in certain areas of the brain** (i.e., hypothalamus, anterior commissure, corpus callosum, thalamus).

B. Gender identity

    1. Gender identity is an individual's **sense of being male or female.**
        a. This awareness develops between 2 and 3 years of age (see Chapter 1).
        b. Gender identity is affected by genetic and hormonal alterations (Table 18-1).

    2. **Gender role** is the expression of gender identity in society.

    3. In **gender identity disorder,** commonly called **transsexuality,** a person feels that he or she was born into the wrong body and may seek sex-change surgery.

C. Sexual orientation

 Patient snapshot 18-2. A 16-year-old boy tells his family physician that he thinks he is gay. He reveals that he has a "platonic" girlfriend, but all of his sexual fantasies and dreams are about men. He then asks the physician if he is "normal."

What is the physician's best response? (see I C 2)

    1. Sexual orientation is the persistent and unchanging **preference for members of one's own sex (homosexuality) or the opposite sex (heterosexuality)** for love and sexual expression.

    2. The *Diagnostic and Statistical Manual of Mental Disorders,* 4th edition (**DSM-**

Table 18-1

Physiologic Abnormalities of Sexual Development

Syndrome	Genotype	Phenotype	Characteristics
Androgen insensitivity (testicular feminization)	XY	Female	• Body cells unresponsive to androgen • Testicles may appear at puberty as labial or inguinal masses
Congenital adrenal hyperplasia (adrenogenital syndrome)	XX	Female (masculinized genitalia)	• Adrenal gland unable to produce adequate cortisone, leading to excessive perinatal adrenal androgen secretion • One third have a lesbian sexual orientation
Turner syndrome	XO	Female	• Fibrous, nonfunctioning ovaries • Short stature and webbed neck

IV), considers **homosexuality** a **normal variant** of sexual expression, not a dysfunction.

3. Estimates of the occurrence of homosexuality are **3% to 10% in men** and **1% to 5% in women.** No significant ethnic differences are found.

4. Cross-gender behavior during childhood may be predictive of later homosexual orientation. This tendency is stronger in boys than in girls.

5. Evidence of **hormonal and genetic influences** on homosexuality include:
  a. Alterations in levels of **prenatal hormones** (i.e., high levels of androgen in female fetuses and decreased levels of androgen in male fetuses). Hormone levels in adulthood are normal.
  b. A **higher concordance rate in monozygotic twins** than in dizygotic twins and genetic markers on the **X chromosome**

6. Because homosexuality is not a dysfunction, **no psychological treatment is needed.** If needed, psychological intervention helps a person who is uncomfortable with his or her sexual orientation to become more comfortable.

II. THE BIOLOGY OF SEXUALITY IN ADULTHOOD

A. Hormones and behavior in women

  1. Estrogen is only minimally involved in **libido,** and therefore **menopause** (i.e., cessation of ovarian estrogen production) and **aging** do not reduce sex drive.

  2. Testosterone is secreted by the adrenal glands throughout adult life and is believed to play an important role in **sex drive** in women as well as in men.

  3. Progesterone, which is contained in many **oral contraceptives,** may inhibit sexual interest and behavior in women.

B. Hormones and behavior in men

  1. Stress may **decrease testosterone levels.**

  2. Medical treatment with **estrogens, progesterone, or antiandrogens** (e.g., to treat prostate cancer) ultimately leads to decreased androgen production, resulting in reduced sexual interest and behavior.

C. The sexual response cycle

    1. Masters and Johnson devised a **four-stage** model for sexual response in both men and women (Table 18-2).

    2. The stages are **excitement, plateau, orgasm and resolution.**

III. SEXUAL DYSFUNCTION AND PARAPHILIAS

Patient snapshot 18-3. A 46-year-old man tells his physician that he is having difficulty gaining erections and would like to have a prescription for Viagra (sildenafil citrate). He then asks the physician how the drug will work to improve his erections.

How best can the physician describe the action of Viagra to this patient? (see III B 2 a)

A. **Sexual dysfunction** involves problems in one or more stages of the sexual response cycle. Categories of sexual dysfunction are shown in Table 18-3.

B. **Treatment.** There is a growing tendency for **physicians to treat the sexual problems of patients** rather than refer these patients to specialists.

    1. **Behavioral treatment** includes the following techniques:

Table 18-2
The Sexual Response Cycle

Men	Women	Both Men and Women
Excitement Stage		
• Penile erection	• Clitoral erection • Labial swelling • Vaginal lubrication • Tenting effect (rising of the uterus in the pelvic cavity)	• Increased pulse, blood pressure, and respiration • Nipple erection
Plateau Stage		
• Increased size and upward movement of the testes • Secretion of a few drops of sperm-containing fluid	• Contraction of the outer one third of the vagina, forming the orgasmic platform (enlargement of the upper one third of the vagina)	• Further increase in pulse, blood pressure, and respiration • Flushing of the chest and face
Orgasm Stage		
• Forcible expulsion of seminal fluid	• Contractions of the uterus and vagina	• Contractions of the anal sphincter
Resolution Stage		
• Refractory, or resting, period in which restimulation is not possible • Length of this period varies by age and physical condition	• Little or no refractory period	• Muscle relaxation • Return of the sexual and cardiovascular systems to the prestimulated state over 10–15 minutes

Table 18-3

DSM-IV Categories of Sexual Dysfunction

Disorder	Characteristics
Hypoactive sexual desire	• Decreased interest in sexual activity
Sexual aversion disorder	• Aversion to and avoidance of sexual activity
Female sexual arousal disorder	• Inability to maintain vaginal lubrication until the sex act is completed, despite adequate physical stimulation • Reported in as many as 20% of women
Male erectile disorder (commonly called impotence)	• Lifelong or primary (rare): Has never had an erection sufficient for penetration • Acquired or secondary (common)*: Current inability to maintain erections despite normal erections in the past • Situational (common): Difficulty maintaining erections in some situations, but not all
Orgasmic disorder (male and female)	• Lifelong: Has never had an orgasm • Acquired: Current inability to achieve orgasm despite adequate genital stimulation and normal orgasms in the past • Reported more often in more women than in men
Premature ejaculation	• Ejaculation before the man wishes • Short or absent plateau phase • Usually accompanied by anxiety • Second most common of all male sexual disorders
Vaginismus	• Painful spasm of the outer one third of the vagina making intercourse or pelvic examination difficult • Vaginal dilators and psychological counseling used for treatment
Dyspareunia	• Persistent pain associated with sexual intercourse • Much more common in women, but can occur in men

DSM-IV = *Diagnostic and Statistical Manual of Mental Disorders,* 4th edition.
*Acquired or secondary erectile disorder is the most common of all male sexual disorders.

    a. Sensate-focus exercise. In this exercise, the individual's awareness of touch, sight, smell, and sound stimuli are increased during sexual activity, and pressure to achieve an erection or orgasm is decreased.

    b. Squeeze technique. This technique is used to treat **premature ejaculation.** The man is taught to identify the sensation that occurs just before the emission phase, when ejaculation can no longer be prevented. At this moment, the man asks his partner to exert pressure on the coronal ridge of the glans on both sides of the penis until the erection subsides, thereby delaying ejaculation.

    c. Relaxation techniques, hypnosis, and systematic desensitization are used to reduce anxiety associated with sexual performance.

    d. Masturbation may be recommended (particularly for orgasmic disorders) to help the patient learn what stimuli are most effective.

  2. Medical and surgical treatments for erectile dysfunction

    a. Sildenafil citrate (Viagra) is used to treat **erectile dysfunction.** It works by blocking the enzyme phosphodiester (PDE) 5, which destroys cyclic guanosine monophosphate (cGMP), a vasodilator that is secreted in the penis with sexual stimulation. Thus, degradation of cGMP is slowed and the erection persists.

    b. Apomorphine (**Uprima**) is a drug that increases the availability of **dopamine,**

a sexually stimulating neurotransmitter, in the brain. It is being used to treat erectile disorder and female arousal disorder. It is dissolved under the tongue and is effective in about 50% of patients.

    c. **Intracorporeal injection of vasodilators (e.g. phentolamine, papaverine)** or implantation of prosthetic devices are also used to treat erectile dysfunction.

C. **Paraphilias,** which occur almost exclusively in men, involve the preferential use of **unusual objects of sexual desire or unusual sexual activities** (Table 18-4).

IV. SPECIAL ISSUES IN SEXUALITY: ILLNESS, INJURY, PREGNANCY, AND AGING

A. Myocardial infarction (MI)

    1. After an MI, many patients experience **erectile dysfunction and decreased libido.** These problems are caused by fear that sexual activity will lead to another heart attack.

    2. Most patients who can tolerate exercise that increases the heart rate to **110 to 130 bpm** (exertion equal to climbing two flights of stairs) can resume sexual activity.

    3. Sexual positions that produce the least exertion for the patient (e.g., the partner in the superior position) are safest following MI.

B. Diabetes

    1. **Erectile dysfunction** is common in diabetic men; orgasm and ejaculation are less likely to be affected.

    2. The major causes of erectile problems in men with diabetes are:
        a. **Diabetic neuropathy,** which involves microscopic damage to nerve tissue in the penis as a result of hyperglycemia
        b. **Vascular changes** that affect the blood vessels in the penis

    3. **Good metabolic control** of diabetes improves erectile function.

C. Spinal cord injuries

    1. In **men,** spinal cord injury causes erectile and orgasmic dysfunction, retrograde ejaculation (into the bladder), reduced testosterone levels, and decreased fertility.

Table 18-4
Sexual Paraphilias

Type	Source of Sexual Gratification
Pedophilia (most common)	Children (under age 14 years); perpetrator must be at least 16 years old and 5 years older than the victim
Exhibitionism	Exposing the genitals to strangers
Sexual masochism and sadism	Receiving (masochism) or causing (sadism) physical suffering or humiliation
Fetishism	Inanimate objects (i.e., rubber, women's shoes)
Frotteurism	Rubbing the penis against a nonconsenting, unaware woman
Necrophilia	Corpses
Transvestic fetishism	Wearing women's underclothing (exclusive to heterosexual men)
Voyeurism	Secretly observing people undressing or engaging in sexual activity

2. The effects of spinal cord injury in **women** have not been well studied. Vaginal lubrication, pelvic vasocongestion, and the incidence of orgasm may be reduced, but fertility does not appear to be adversely affected.

D. Pregnancy

1. **An increased sex drive** may occur in some pregnant women, possibly associated with **pelvic vasocongestion.**

2. **A decreased sex drive** is more common and is caused by physical discomfort, the association of motherhood with decreased sexual attractiveness, or fear of harming the fetus.

3. Many obstetricians suggest **cessation of sexual intercourse approximately 4 weeks before the expected date of delivery.** This may place a strain on a marriage.

E. **Aging.** Most men and women continue to have sexual interest as they age.

1. In **men,** physical changes include the need for more direct genital stimulation, slower erection, diminished intensity of ejaculation, and an increased refractory period.

2. In **women,** physical changes include vaginal thinning, shortening of vaginal length, and vaginal dryness. These changes can be reversed with **estrogen replacement therapy.**

V. DRUGS AND SEXUALITY

A. **Prescription drugs.** Antihypertensives, antidepressants, antipsychotics, and other agents affect libido, erection, orgasm, and ejaculation, often as a result of their effects on neurotransmitter systems (Table 18-5).

B. **Drugs of abuse** also affect sexuality (Table 18-6).

Table 18-5
Neurotransmitters and Sexual Response

Neurotransmitter (Representative Drug) ($\uparrow$ increased availability, $\downarrow$ decreased availability)	Sexual Function ($\uparrow$ enhanced, $\downarrow$ inhibited)
$\uparrow$ Serotonin (fluoxetine; trazodone)	$\downarrow$ Orgasm and ejaculation; SSRIs are used to treat premature ejaculation; trazodone can cause priapism
$\uparrow$ Dopamine (levodopa, apomorphine)	$\uparrow$ Libido and erection
$\downarrow$ Dopamine (chlorpromazine)	$\downarrow$ Erection
$\downarrow$ Norepinephrine β (propranolol)	$\downarrow$ Erection
$\uparrow$ Norepinephrine α_2 in the periphery (yohimbine)	$\uparrow$ Erection

SSRI = selective serotonin reuptake inhibitor.

Table 18-6
The Effects of Drugs of Abuse on Sexuality

Drug	Effect
Alcohol	• Acute use: Increased libido because of psychological disinhibition, erectile dysfunction • Chronic use: Erectile dysfunction due to increased estrogen availability as a result of liver damage
Marijuana	• Acute use: Increased libido because of psychological disinhibition • Chronic use: Reduced testosterone levels in men and lowered pituitary gonadotropin levels in women
Amphetamines and cocaine	• Increased libido because of enhancement of dopaminergic effects on the brain
Heroin and methadone	• Reduced libido and inhibited ejaculation • Fewer problems with methadone

Answers to Patient Snapshot Questions

18-1. The most likely diagnosis for this patient is androgen insensitivity syndrome (testicular feminization). Patients with this condition are males with a genetic defect in which the body cells do not respond to androgen produced by the testes. External genitalia are feminine and the testicles, which descend at puberty, may appear as labial or inguinal masses.

18-2. The physician's best response is to reassure this young man that he is normal. The young man may or may not be homosexual; like heterosexuality, homosexuality is a normal variant of sexual expression.

18-3. Sildenafil citrate (Viagra) works by blocking phosphodiester (PDE) 5, which destroys cyclic guanosine monophosphate (cGMP), which is secreted in the penis with sexual stimulation. Degradation of cGMP, a vasodilator, is slowed and the erection persists.

19

Aggression and Abuse

 Patient snapshot 19-1. A 25-year-old man is brought to the emergency room after being injured in a fight, which he provoked at a football game. The patient, who is a bodybuilder, denies that he has been drinking or taking drugs. The patient tells the doctor, "I am taking my orders directly from heaven."

Given this clinical picture, what is the most likely cause of this man's behavior? (see I B 1 b)

I. AGGRESSION

A. Social determinants of aggression

1. **Homicide,** which occurs more often in **low socioeconomic groups,** is increasing. At least 50% of homicides are committed with **guns.**

2. Children who are likely to become violent adults often have the following characteristics:
   a. High levels of aggression and antisocial behavior (e.g., starting fires, truancy)
   b. Cruelty to animals
   c. Low intelligence quotient (IQ) and poor school grades
   d. Inability to defer gratification
   e. Physical or sexual abuse by parents or other caregivers

3. **Violence on television** correlates directly with increased aggression in children.

B. Biologic determinants

1. Androgens
   a. Androgens are closely associated with aggression. **Males are more aggressive than females** in most animal species and human societies.
   b. Bodybuilders who take **androgenic or anabolic steroids** to increase muscle mass may show increased aggression and even psychosis. Withdrawal may cause severe depression.

2. **Drugs.** While intoxicated, heroin users show little aggression. Increased aggression is associated with the use of **alcohol, cocaine, amphetamines, phencyclidine (PCP),** and extremely **high doses of marijuana.**

3. **Serotonin and γ-aminobutyric acid (GABA) inhibit** aggression. **Dopamine and norepinephrine increase** aggression.

4. Abnormalities of the brain (i.e., abnormal activity in the amygdala and prepiriform area; psychomotor and temporal lobe epilepsy) and lesions of the temporal lobe, frontal lobe, and hypothalamus are associated with increased aggression.

Violent people often have a history of **head injury** and show abnormal electroencephalogram (EEG) readings.

II. ABUSE AND NEGLECT OF CHILDREN AND THE ELDERLY

Patient snapshot 19-2. An 82-year-old man is brought to the emergency room by his daughter with whom he lives. The patient seems confused and is unable to tell the physician what year it is or the name of the President of the United States. Physical examination reveals abrasions on one wrist and a spiral fracture of the radius of the other arm. When asked about his injuries, the patient says that he "fell."

What is the physician's next step? (see II B 1)

A. Characteristics and incidence

1. **Child abuse and elder abuse** include:

a. **Physical abuse.** The characteristics of the abused and abuser and signs of abuse are listed in Tables 19-1 and 19-2.

b. **Sexual abuse.** Although relatively rare, sexual abuse does occur in the elderly; signs include abnormal vaginal bleeding and genital bruising. Signs of sexual abuse in children are listed in Table 19-3.

c. **Emotional abuse.** In children, this includes physical neglect as well as rejection by parents or withholding of parental love and attention. In the elderly, neglect of needed care and exploitation for monetary gain are seen.

2. Reported child and elder abuse are **increasing** in the United States; although many cases are not reported, at least **1 million cases of each** are currently reported.

B. Role of the physician

1. If child or elder neglect or physical or sexual abuse is suspected, the **physician must report the case to the appropriate social service agency** and, if necessary, admit the abused to the hospital to ensure his or her safety.

Table 19-1
Child and Elder Physical Abuse: Characteristics of the Abused and the Abuser

Category	Child Abuse	Elder abuse
Characteristics of the abuser	• Substance abuse • Poverty and social isolation • Closest family member (e.g., mother, father) is most likely to abuse • Personal history of victimization by caretaker or spouse	• Substance abuse • Poverty and social isolation • Closest family member (e.g., spouse, daughter, son, or other relative with whom the elder lives and is often financially supported by) is most likely to abuse
Characteristics of the abused	• Prematurity, low birth weight • Hyperactivity or mild physical handicap • Perception of the child as "slow" or "different" • Colicky or "fussy" infant • Most are younger than 5 years of age (33% of cases); 25% of cases are age 5 to 9	• Some degree of dementia • Physical dependence on others • Does not report the abuse, but instead says that he injured himself

Table 19-2
Signs of Abuse

Sign	Child Abuse	Elder Abuse
Neglect	• Poor personal care (e.g., diaper rash, dirty hair) • Lack of needed nutrition	• Poor personal care (e.g., urine odor in incontinent person) • Lack of needed nutrition • Lack of medication or health aids (e.g., eyeglasses, dentures)
Bruises	• Particularly in areas not likely to be injured during normal play, such as buttocks or lower back • Belt or belt buckle marks	• Often bilateral and often on the arms caused by being grabbed
Fractures and burns	• Fractures at different stages of healing • Spiral fractures caused by twisting the limbs • Cigarette burns • Burns on the feet or buttocks due to immersion in hot water	• Fractures at different stages of healing • Spiral fractures caused by twisting the limbs • Cigarette and other burns

Table 19-3
Sexual Abuse of Children

Occurrence	• At least 250,000 cases are reported annually • Reported more now than in the past • Approximately 25% of all girls and 12% of all boys report sexual abuse at some time during their lives
Characteristics of the abuser	• Most are male and known to the child (e.g., uncle, father, mother's boyfriend, family acquaintance) • Alcohol and drug use • Marital problems or no appropriate alternate sexual partner • May be a pedophile
Characteristics of the abused	• Most are 9 to 12 years of age • 25% are younger than 8 years of age • Fear of withdrawal of affection or retribution from the abuser if the abuse is revealed • Shame and inappropriate guilt
Physical signs of abuse	• STDs; children do not contract STDs through casual contact with an infected person or from bedclothes, towels, or toilet seats • Genital or anal injury • Recurrent urinary tract infections
Psychological signs of abuse	• Specific knowledge about sexual acts (e.g., fellatio) in a young child; children have only a vague knowledge about sexual activities • There may be no physical findings in cases not involving penetration • Excessive initiation of sexual activity with friends

STDs = sexually transmitted diseases.

2. The physician is **not required to tell the suspected child or elder abuser** that she suspects abuse, and does not need family consent to hospitalize the abused child or elderly person for protection or treatment.

III. PHYSICAL AND SEXUAL ABUSE OF DOMESTIC PARTNERS

A. Overview

    1. Domestic abuse is a **common** reason for young and middle-aged women to visit the hospital emergency room. Bruises, blackened eyes, and broken bones are often seen.

    2. A woman's risk of being killed by her abuser is greatly increased if she leaves him.

    3. **Characteristics of abusers and abused partners** are listed in Table 19-4.

B. Role of the physician

    1. In contrast to physical or sexual abuse of a child or elderly person, direct reporting by the physician of domestic partner abuse is not appropriate because the victim is usually a competent adult.

    2. A physician who suspects domestic abuse should **provide emotional support** to the abused partner, refer her to an appropriate shelter or program, and **encourage her to report** the case to law enforcement officials.

IV. SEXUAL AGGRESSION: RAPE AND RELATED CRIMES

A. Definitions

    1. **Rape** is a crime of violence, not of passion. Rape is known legally as **sexual assault** or **aggravated sexual assault.**

    2. **Sodomy** is **oral or anal penetration.** The victim may be male or female.

    3. Characteristics of rape, the rapist, and the victim are listed in Table 19-5.

B. Legal considerations

    1. **Rapists may use condoms** to avoid contracting HIV, to avoid DNA identification. Because rapists may have difficulty with erection or ejaculation, semen may not be present in the vagina of a rape victim.

Table 19-4
Physical and Sexual Abuse of Domestic Partners

Characteristics of the abuser	• Is almost always male • Often uses alcohol or drugs • Is impulsive and angry • Has a low tolerance for frustration • Has threatened to kill the abused if she reports or leaves him • Shows apologetic and loving behavior after the abuse • Has low self-esteem
Characteristics of the abused	• Is financially or emotionally dependent on the abuser • Is often pregnant (injuries are often in the "baby zone," i.e., the breasts and abdomen) • Blames herself for the abuse • May neither report to the police nor leave the abuser • Has low self-esteem

Table 19-5
Rape

Definition	• Sexual contact without consent involving vaginal penetration by a penis, finger, or object • Erection and ejaculation do not have to occur
Characteristics of the rapist	• Usually younger than age 25 • Usually the same race as the victim • Usually known by the victim • Alcohol use
Characteristics of the victim	• Usually between 16 and 24 years of age • Usually occurs inside the victim's home • Vaginal injuries may be absent, particularly in parous women (those who have had children)
Characteristics of the crime	• Most rapes are not reported; only 25% are reported to the police • Others tend to blame the victim (e.g., for wearing provocative clothing or for going out at night)
Recovery	• The emotional recovery period commonly lasts at least 1 year • Posttraumatic stress disorder may occur (see Chapter 14) • Group therapy with other rape victims is most effective

2. A victim is **not required to prove that she resisted the rapist** for him to be convicted.

3. In almost every state, **husbands can be prosecuted for raping their wives.** It is illegal to force anyone to engage in sexual activity.

4. Statutory rape. Consensual sex may be considered rape if the victim is younger than 16 or 18 years old (depending on state law) or is **mentally handicapped.**

C. Role of the physician

1. The physician is not required to notify the police if the woman is a competent adult. As in cases of domestic abuse (see III B), the physician should **encourage the patient to notify the police.**

2. The physician should **be supportive and nonjudgmental** during the history and physical examination and should not question the patient's veracity or judgment.

Answers to Patient Snapshot Questions

19-1. It is likely that this bodybuilder has been taking anabolic steroids. In addition to increasing aggressiveness, these agents may cause psychotic symptoms (e.g., the belief that his behavior is being directed from heaven).

19-2. It is likely that this elderly, demented patient has been physically abused, probably by his daughter. The physician's next step is to notify the appropriate social service agency and to protect the patient until the agency takes over the case.

20

The Physician–Patient Relationship

I. COMMUNICATING WITH PATIENTS

 Patient snapshot 20-1. A 5-year-old girl needs to have a procedure that involves minor pain. In the physician's presence, the child's father tells her that it will not hurt.

What should the physician say to the child and the father? (see I A 3)

A. Responding to patients' behavior and questions

  1. Physicians are responsible for dealing with the questions and behavioral problems of their patients. **Referral to other physicians should be reserved for medical problems** outside of the range of the treating physician.

  2. **Adult patients** generally **are told the complete truth** about the diagnosis and prognosis of their illness.
    a. Falsely reassuring or patronizing statements are not used.
    b. Information about the illness is given directly to the adult patient and **not relayed through relatives.**

  3. Children should also be told the truth about their illness or the discomfort of treatment in a way that they can understand. However, parents have the ultimate choice as to whether, when, and how much to tell a child who is ill.

  4. Tables 20-1 and 20-2 provide information about common **USMLE questions** that require students to choose the correct verbal response to a patient's query or action (students often refer to these questions as **the "quote" questions**).

B. Getting information from patients

  1. **Communication and interviewing skills.** During a clinical interview, a physician must establish a relationship (rapport), **gain the patient's trust,** and then gather physical, psychological, and social information to identify the patient's problem.

  2. Interviewing techniques
    a. **Direct questions** are used to elicit information quickly in an emergency situation (e.g., "Have you been shot?") or when the **patient is seductive** or overly talkative.
    b. **Open-ended questions** are used to obtain as much information as possible and **encourage the patient to speak freely** (e.g., "What brought you to the hospital today?").
    c. Table 20-3 lists interviewing techniques that are useful in communicating with patients.

Table 20-1
The USMLE "Quote" Questions: Emotional Issues

	What the Physician Should Say to the Patient (or Relative)
Angry, complaining, and seductive patients	
A 40-year-old male patient snaps at you about the amount of time that he had to sit in the waiting room.	"I apologize. It must be hard to have to wait so long." Show support for the way the patient must feel. Do not take his anger personally. He is probably fearful about becoming dependent as well as of being ill.
A 50-year-old, dirty, disheveled patient has had at least one complaint about the office or staff on every visit. Today she complains that one of your best nurses was "fresh" to her.	"I will speak to the nurse about what happened." Do not blame the patient, no matter how provocative he or she is, for problems with the office staff.
A 28-year-old male patient comes up close to you and tells you that he finds you attractive.	"Let's talk about the problem that brought you here." Romantic relationships with patients are never appropriate. Gather information using direct rather than open-ended questions, set limits on the behavior that you will tolerate, and use a chaperone when interviewing and examining the patient.
A 38-year-old cancer patient complains to you about the way one of her other physicians spoke to her.	"It is a good idea to speak to your other physician directly about your concerns." Do not intervene in the patient's relationship with the other physician unless there is a medical reason to do so.
A 40-year-old male patient with pneumonia insists on having a CAT scan, which the physician knows he does not need.	"Tell me why you want the CAT scan." Find out why the patient wants the CAT scan, and try to address his underlying concerns. Do not perform a procedure that you know is unnecessary.
Noncompliant patients	
A 45-year-old patient whose parents both died of colon cancer before age 50 refuses to have a colonoscopy because she heard that the procedure was uncomfortable.	"Tell me your concerns about the procedure." Identify the real reason for the patient's refusal (e.g., fear that cancer will be found). Do not attempt to scare the patient into complying (e.g., providing photographs of untreated cases).
A 68-year-old female patient insists on stopping a needed treatment (e.g., wants her pacemaker removed or wants to stop chemotherapy) because it is making her uncomfortable.	"Let's discuss ways that we can make the treatment more tolerable for you." Do not stop treatment before you have explored the alternatives.
A nurse tells you that she saw a hospitalized 55-year-old patient with diabetes putting sugar in her coffee.	"Let's discuss your diet again." Do not become angry at noncompliant patients. This patient may need to be reminded of how to follow her diet.
A patient believes (falsely) that his poor health behavior (e.g., smoking) is actually beneficial to his health.	"How do you feel about your cigarette smoking?" Do not recommend methods of smoking cessation until the patient is willing to try to stop.

(*continued*)

Table 20-1—*Continued*
The USMLE "Quote" Questions: Emotional Issues

	What the Physician Should Say to the Patient (or Relative)
Depressed and anxious patients	
A 48-year-old married woman who had a mastectomy says she feels "ugly" when she gets undressed at night.	"Tell me about your relationship with your husband." Find out why the patient feels this way. Do not offer falsely reassuring statements like "you still look good."
Without telling you what he is feeling, a 54-year-old hypertensive patient asks you to tell him more about his illness and the side effects of medication he is taking.	"Tell me exactly what you are experiencing now." This patient may be reluctant to bring up embarrassing issues associated with the illness or treatment (e.g., sexual problems).
A 45-year-old woman has an illness that has caused skin lesions. She asks you how she should deal with the negative reactions of other people.	"Let's come up with something that you can say to a person who has a reaction that bothers you." Then work with her to devise a statement such as, "I had an illness that caused some skin problems, but it is not contagious."
A 44-year-old AIDS patient tells you that he will kill himself when he gets out of the hospital.	"I would like you to remain in the hospital for a few more days." Do not release a patient who has made a serious suicidal threat. If the patient refuses to stay you can hold him involuntarily for a period of time. (see Chapter 15)

Table 20-2
The USMLE "Quote" Questions: Developmental Issues

	What the Physician Should Say to the Patient (or Relative)
Child and adolescent patients	
A 9-year-old child with leukemia asks you what is wrong with him. His parents have told you that they do not want him to know he has leukemia.	"What have your parents told you about your illness?" Only the parents of ill children decide what to tell the child about the illness. With the parents' permission, you may present the information to the child in the most supportive and nonthreatening way possible.
The parents of a 15-year-old girl want you to tell her to give up her newborn child for adoption. The girl wants to keep the baby.	"If you decide to keep the child, these are the things that you can expect that the child will need from you as he grows up." Provide information to the teenager about the practical issues of what the baby will need throughout its childhood. Do not make decisions for the family regarding adoption. If they ask, it is appropriate to tell them about the options.
Reproductive issues for patients	
A couple with five children would like to use sterilization for birth control. They ask you whether they should choose a tubal ligation or a vasectomy.	"Here are the pros and cons of each procedure; think about them and let me know what you decide." Do not make medical decisions for patients, and do not get involved in the issue of which partner will have the procedure. Give them all of the relevant information and let them decide on a course of action.

(continued)

Table 20-2—*Continued*
The USMLE "Quote" Questions: Developmental Issues

	What the Physician Should Say to the Patient (or Relative)

Reproductive issues for patients

The parents of a healthy, mentally retarded, pregnant 17 year old want you to perform an abortion. The girl wants to keep the baby whom tests have shown has Down syndrome.	"Because the patient does not want an abortion, I cannot do it." Do not recommend a course of action (e.g., adoption), but do facilitate discussion about the options between the parents and the patient. The fact that the baby has Down syndrome is irrelevant.
A 25-year-old patient requests a first-trimester abortion from a physician who has religious and moral prohibitions against abortion.	"I do not perform abortions, but I will refer you to a doctor who does." You are not required to perform any procedure a patient requests. Do not be judgmental, do not impose your own beliefs on the patient, and do not try to change her mind.

Elderly and dying patients

An 82-year-old woman has had two falls at home. She tells you that her adult children are concerned and want her to go into a nursing home. She does not want to go.	"Let's try to find out why you are falling." Conduct a medical evaluation and a home evaluation to determine why the patient is falling. Then treat her medical problems and recommend environmental changes (e.g., remove area rugs to prevent tripping), which will allow her to stay safely at home as long as possible.
A 60-year-old dying patient asks you how long he has to live. You know that he is likely to live about three months.	"While there have been exceptions, most people at this stage of the illness live about three months." Be truthful, direct, and kind. Reassure the patient that you will not abandon him, but do not offer philosophical or religious statements.
A 76-year-old male patient, who is of a different religion than you are, tells you that he had a religious "vision" while praying and asks you to pray with him.	"That must have been a very important moment for you." Although you do not have to pray with the patient, you should show support and understanding of his belief system.
The brother of a 60-year-old competent woman who has terminal lung cancer asks you her diagnosis and prognosis.	"Please ask your sister." Do not discuss issues concerning patients with their relatives or anyone else without the patient's permission.

II. THE ILL PATIENT

A. Seeking medical and psychiatric care

   1. Only about **one third of individuals with physical symptoms seek medical care;** most people treat themselves at home using over-the-counter medications.

   2. Patients with psychiatric symptoms are even less likely to seek help.

      a. In the United States, there is a **stigma attached to having psychological problems;** they are considered an indication of "moral weakness" or lack of self-control.

      b. Psychiatric illness is strongly associated with physical illness. **Morbidity and mortality rates** are much higher in patients who need psychiatric care.

Table 20-3
Interviewing Techniques

Patient snapshot. The emergency squad brings a 75-year-old man to the hospital after a fall. While taking a brief history, the physician notes that the patient seems frightened and in pain. The patient says that he is "fine" and just wants to go home.

How can the physician use the clinical interview to find out what this patient is experiencing now?

Technique	Example
Aim: To establish rapport by expressing interest, understanding, and concern, and by giving value and credence to the patient's feelings	
Support and empathy	"That fall must have been a frightening experience for you."
Validation	"Many people would feel scared if they had been injured as you were."
Aim: To maximize information-gathering by encouraging the patient to elaborate on an answer	
Facilitation	"Please tell me what happened."
Reflection	"You said that your pain increased during the ambulance trip?"
Silence	The physician waits in silence for the patient to speak.
Aim: To clarify information by calling the patient's attention to inconsistencies in his responses or body language, and by summarizing the information obtained during the interview	
Confrontation	"You say that you feel fine but you seem to be in pain."
Recapitulation	"Let's go over what happened this morning. You fell in the shower and hurt your leg. You could not move it, so your wife called the emergency squad. The paramedics brought you to the hospital. Have I gotten it right?"

B. The "sick role." A sick person assumes a specific role in society and follows predictable behavioral patterns (i.e., the "sick role," described by Parsons). These patterns include **exemption** from usual responsibilities, **expectation of care** by others, **efforts** toward getting better, and **cooperation** with health care personnel.

C. Defense mechanisms, such as denial (i.e., refusal to admit to being sick; see Chapter 4), may help patients to cope with the initial phase of serious illness. Over the long term, such defense mechanisms can cause a delay in seeking treatment and this may prove harmful.

III. COMPLIANCE

Patient snapshot 20-2. A physician becomes very angry with her 80-year-old patient when he confesses that he has not been following her recommended diet and activity program. The physician's own father died of congestive heart failure 5 years earlier, and he had never exercised and rarely watched his diet.

What is going on in this physician-patient relationship? (see III B 3)

A. Characteristics

    1. Compliance is the extent to which a patient **follows the instructions** of the physician.

    2. Compliance is **not related** to a patient's gender, religion, socioeconomic or marital status, race, intelligence, or education.

3. Factors that increase and decrease compliance are listed in Table 20-4.

B. Transference reactions. Patients have unconscious reactions to their physicians, which involve a transfer of emotions from childhood parent-child relationships (see Chapter 4). These emotions may affect patient compliance.

1. In **positive transference,** patients view physicians as good and have a high level of confidence in their abilities.

2. In **negative transference,** patients feel excessive resentment or anger toward the physician if the patients' expectations are not met. These patients may not comply with medical advice.

3. Countertransference is the reaction of physicians toward their patients. Physicians may feel guilty when they cannot help a patient, may minimize the severity of illness in a colleague whom they are treating, or may have **positive, negative, or inappropriate feelings toward patients who remind them of close relatives or friends.** All of these can result in the patient not receiving the appropriate care from the physician.

IV. STRESS AND ILLNESS

A. Life stress is associated with both **physical and emotional illness.**

1. Stressful life events may be **negative** (e.g., death of a spouse) or **positive** (e.g., birth of a wanted child).

2. Holmes categorized life stressors according to a **point value system,** with 100 points (e.g., death of a spouse) representing the highest level of stress. Individuals who accumulate 300 points in 1 year may be at risk for serious illness.

Table 20-4
Factors Associated with Compliance with Medical Advice

Factors That Increase Compliance	Factors That Decrease Compliance
Good physician-patient relationship (most important factor)	Perception of the physician as cold and unapproachable; anger at the physician
Feeling ill and limitation of usual activities	Few symptoms and little disruption of activities
Written instructions for taking medication	Verbal instructions for taking medication
Acute illness	Chronic illness
Simple treatment schedule	Complex treatment schedule
Short time spent in the waiting room	Long time spent in the waiting room
Recommending one behavioral change at a time (e.g., "This month, stop smoking.")	Recommending multiple behavioral changes at the same time (e.g., "This month, stop smoking, start exercising, and begin a diet.")
Belief that the benefits of care outweigh its financial and time costs (the "Health Belief Model")	Belief that the financial and time costs of care outweigh its benefits
Peer support (particularly in adolescents with chronic illnesses)	Little peer support

B. Psychosomatic disorders

1. Psychological stress **exacerbates physical disorders** such as congestive heart failure, cardiac arrhythmia, hyperthyroidism, peptic ulcer disease, ulcerative colitis, rheumatoid arthritis, low back pain, tension and migraine headaches, diabetes mellitus, and immune system disorders.

2. The **type A personality** is characterized by **time pressure and competitiveness. Coronary artery disease** is seen more commonly in type A patients who also are **aggressive and hostile.**

3. **Hans Selye** described the stages of the body's response to stress as the **general adaptation syndrome.** Adrenocorticotropic hormone (ACTH) is released rapidly, followed by the release of corticosteroids that suppress immune response.

V. SPECIAL PATIENT POPULATIONS

A. **At-risk patients.** When hospitalized, certain patients are at greater risk for psychological reactions to illness, hospitalization, or surgery. These include:

1. Patients with a **history of psychiatric illness and patients having certain personality styles and disorders** (see Table 14-4)

2. Patients whose **relationships** with their families or with the medical staff worsen during the illness. **Fear** of illness can result in expressions of **anger** toward medical personnel.

3. Patients in the **intensive care unit,** who lack a sense of control of the environment and have few orienting cues

4. Patients receiving **renal dialysis,** because of their dependence on technology and other people for survival

5. **Surgical patients** who have **unrealistic expectations** for a procedure, believe that they will **not survive surgery,** or **deny** that they are seriously worried before surgery
  a. Surgical patients who **express their anxiety** are at lower risk for morbidity and mortality.
  b. The outcome is also improved for surgical patients who **know what to expect** during and after the procedure (e.g., pain, disorientation, mechanical support).

B. Patients with AIDS

1. Common responses to this diagnosis include intense anxiety, hopelessness, depression, and guilt (if their behavior may have led to the disease).

2. Patients require reassurance that **they will not be abandoned** by their physician, family, and friends.

C. Chronic pain patients

1. **Chronic pain** is common and may be caused by **psychological or physical factors,** or both. A good physician-patient relationship is an important part of the treatment of chronic pain.

2. **Psychosocial factors** associated with chronic pain include **depression,** neglect, physical and sexual **abuse** in childhood, and life **stress.**

3. **Scheduled administration of medication** is more effective than medication administered on demand, because scheduled administration separates the experience of pain from the receipt of medication. Medication given on demand links the two.

4. Many patients with chronic pain are **undermedicated.**

   a. Patients may be undermedicated because the physician fears that the patient will become addicted to the medication.

   b. However, recent evidence shows that patients with chronic pain **do not become addicted** to opiate drugs. Unlike addicts, these patients easily discontinue the use of drugs as the pain remits.

5. According to the **gate control theory,** the perception of pain can be blocked by electric stimulation of large-diameter afferent nerves. Some patients are helped by this treatment.

6. **Pain tolerance** can be increased through biofeedback, physical therapy, hypnosis, psychotherapy, meditation, and relaxation training.

Answers to Patient Snapshot Questions

20-1. The physician should not contradict the father in front of the child. However, the physician should take the father aside and advise him that children, like adults, need to be told the truth about what to expect from a medical procedure. With the father's consent, the doctor should then tell the child about how much pain she is likely to feel in a way that she will understand (e.g., "This will feel like a bug bite").

20-2. This physician who becomes angry at her patient for failing to comply with her recommendations is showing a countertransference reaction. This show of emotion is a result of unconsciously reexperiencing feelings about her own father in her current relationship with the patient.

21

Health Care Delivery

Patient snapshot 21-1. An 89-year-old man with a spinal compression fracture is brought to the hospital by ambulance. After a 7-day hospital stay, the patient is moved to a nursing facility for rehabilitation. After 1 month in the nursing facility, it is determined that the patient cannot care for himself and will need long-term nursing home care.

How will this patient's medical bills—ie, ambulance, hospital bills, rehabilitation facility, and nursing home bills—be paid? (see Table 21-1)

I. HEALTH CARE DELIVERY SYSTEMS

A. Hospitals

1. Surplus. The United States has over 6000 hospitals and 1,000,000 hospital beds. The current surplus of hospital beds is partly due to restrictions on length of hospital stays imposed by insurance companies.

2. Types of hospitals
   a. Voluntary hospitals. Most hospitals in the United States are owned privately or sponsored by churches, universities, or community governments. These institutions are not for profit.
   b. Investor-owned hospitals represent about 12% of all hospitals. These for-profit ventures may be oriented to general or specialty care.
   c. Veteran's Administration and **military hospitals** are owned and operated by the **federal government.**
   d. Long-term psychiatric hospitals usually are owned and operated by state governments.
   e. Municipal hospitals are owned and operated by city governments. These institutions are often teaching hospitals affiliated with medical schools.

B. **Nursing homes.** The United States currently has about 25,000 nursing homes that **provide long-term care,** particularly for the elderly.

1. Nursing homes are classified according to the **level of care** that they offer. Costs of nursing home care range from about $35,000 per year for residential facilities that provide limited nursing care to $75,000 per year for skilled nursing care facilities.

2. Only about **5%** of the elderly utilize long-term nursing home care. **Most** elderly Americans spend the last years of life **in their own residences.**

C. Hospices

1. Hospices use physicians, nurses, social workers, and volunteers to provide **inpa-**

tient and outpatient supportive care to **terminally ill patients** (i.e., those expected to live < 6 months).

2. Hospices offer patients **death with dignity** and **as little pain as possible.** They provide grief counseling, peer and family support, and administration of pain medication as needed.

II. PHYSICIANS

A. Medical specialization

1. The United States currently has **approximately 650,000 physicians.**

2. **Primary care physicians,** including family practitioners, internists, and pediatricians, provide initial care to patients and account for one third of all physicians. This number is increasing and is expected to soon reach one half of all physicians. **The number of specialists is decreasing.**

B. Patient consultations

1. In the United States, people average **five visits to physicians per year,** significantly fewer visits than people in developed countries with systems of socialized medicine.

2. For high-income patients, most physician-patient contact occurs in a physician's office. Low-income patients are more likely to seek treatment in hospital outpatient departments.

3. The **most common reasons for physician visits** are upper respiratory ailments and injuries.

III. COST OF HEALTH CARE

A. Health care expenditures

1. Health care expenditures in the United States total more than **15% of the gross domestic product (GDP),** more than in any other industrialized society.

2. Health care expenditures have increased because of the **increasing age of the population,** advances in medical technology, and the availability of health care to the poor and elderly through Medicaid and Medicare, respectively (see IV D).

B. Allocation of health care funds

1. **Hospitalization is the most expensive element** of health care in the United States. Physician costs are the next most expensive, followed by the cost of nursing homes, medications and medical supplies, mental health services, and dental and other care.

2. **The federal government, state governments,** private health insurance, and individuals each pay about one quarter of all health care costs.

IV. HEALTH INSURANCE

A. Overview

1. The United States is the only industrialized country that **does not have publicly mandated government-funded health care insurance coverage** for all citizens.

2. Certain citizens, such as the **elderly** and the **poor,** do have government-funded health care insurance.

3. Most Americans must **obtain their own health insurance** through their employer or on their own. About 15% of Americans have **no health insurance** and must pay the costs of health care themselves.

B. Private health insurance

1. **Blue Cross/Blue Shield,** a nonprofit private insurance carrier, is regulated by insurance agencies in each state and pays for hospital costs (Blue Cross) and physician fees and diagnostic tests (Blue Shield) for 30%–50% of working people in the United States.

2. Individuals can also contract with one of approximately 1000 other **private insurance carriers,** such as Aetna or Prudential.

3. Most insurance carriers offer a traditional, **fee-for-service** insurance plan and at least one type of managed care plan.

C. Managed care and fee-for-service plans

1. **Managed care** describes a health care delivery system in which all aspects of an individual's health care are coordinated or managed by a group of providers to enhance cost effectiveness.

    a. A managed care plan has **restrictions on provider choice** and referrals and relatively **low premiums.**

    b. Because fewer patient visits result in lower costs, the philosophy of managed care stresses **prevention** rather than acute treatment.

    c. Types of managed care plans include health maintenance organizations **(HMOs),** preferred provider organizations **(PPOs)** and point of service **(POS)** plans. In the more restrictive, less costly plans, there is a "**gatekeeper**" physician who decides if and when a patient needs to see a specialist.

2. A **fee-for-service plan** has **no restrictions on provider choice** or referrals but commonly has **higher premiums.**

D. Federal and state-funded insurance coverage

1. Medicare and Medicaid are government-funded programs that provide medical insurance to certain groups of people (Table 21-1).

2. **Diagnosis-related groups (DRGs)** are used by Medicare to pay hospital bills. The amount paid is based on an estimate of the cost of hospitalization for each illness rather than the actual charges incurred.

3. Two major shortcomings of Medicare are that **it does not cover outpatient prescription drugs or long-term nursing home care.** Elderly patients must pay for these services on their own.

V. DEMOGRAPHICS OF HEALTH

Patient snapshot 21-2. A physician has four patients waiting to see her in the hospital emergency room: two men (one from a low socioeconomic group and one from a high socioeconomic group) and two women (one from a low socioeconomic group and one from a high socioeconomic group).

If the physician were to see the sickest person first, which patient would that probably be? (see V B 2, C 1)

A. Lifestyle, attitudes, and health

1. Lifestyle and poor dietary and other habits (particularly smoking) are responsible for about **70% of physical illness.**

2. **Attitudes** are also important in health. For example, although transplants can save many lives, there are fewer transplant procedures done than are needed. This is

Table 21-1

Medicare and Medicaid

Funding	Eligibility	Coverage
Medicare		
Federal government (through the Social Security system)	• People eligible for social security benefits (e.g., those 65 years of age regardless of income) and people of any age with chronic disabilities or debilitating illnesses	• **Part A:** Inpatient hospital costs, home health care, nursing home care for a limited time after hospitalization (for a maximum of about 3 months), hospice care • **Part B*:** Dialysis, physical therapy, laboratory tests, outpatient hospital care, physician bills, ambulance service, medical equipment
Medicaid (Medical in California)		
Both federal and state governments**	• Indigent (very low income) people • One third of all monies are allocated for nursing home care for indigent, elderly people	• Inpatient and outpatient hospital costs • Physician services • Home health care • Hospice care • Laboratory tests and dialysis • Prescription drugs • Long-term nursing home care

*Part B is optional and has a 20% co-payment and a $100 deductible.
**The state contribution is determined by average per capita income of the state.

primarily because there are **not enough people willing to donate their organs** at death.

B. **Socioeconomic status and health**

    1. Socioeconomic status is based primarily on **occupation,** with secondary emphasis on **educational level;** it is associated also with place of residence and with income.

    2. Because of the costs, people in low socioeconomic groups **delay seeking health care** and are more likely to be very ill when first consulting a physician.

C. **Gender, age, and health**

    1. **Men** are less likely to seek medical care. They are also are more likely to have heart disease and shorter life expectancies than women.

    2. **Women** are at higher risk than men for developing **autoimmune diseases, smoking- and alcohol-related illnesses,** and **AIDS when they are already HIV positive.**

    3. Although the **elderly** comprise only 12% of the population, they currently incur over **30% of all health care costs;** this figure is expected to rise to 50% by the year 2020.

    4. The leading **causes of death** differ by age group (Table 21-2).

Table 21-2

Leading Causes of Death by Age Group*

Age Group	Causes of Death (Approximate Number)
Infants (< 1 year)	• Congenital anomalies (7,100) • Sudden infant death syndrome (SIDS) (4,700) • Respiratory distress syndrome (1,800)
Children (1–4 years)	• Accidents (2,600) • Congenital anomalies (800) • Cancer (primarily leukemia and CNS malignancies) (500)
Children (5–14 years)	• Accidents (3,500) • Cancer (primarily leukemia and CNS malignancies) (1,100) • Homicide and legal intervention (700)
Adolescents/young adults (15–24 years)	• Accidents (most are motor vehicle) (14,000) • Homicide and legal intervention (8,400) • Suicide (4,800)
Adults (25–44 years)	• Accidents (27,300) • HIV infection (27,200) • Cancer (21,900)
Middle-age adults (45–64 years)	• Cancer (133,100) • Heart disease (105,000) • Stroke (14,700)
Elderly (65 and over)	• Heart disease (620,000) • Cancer (in decreasing order: lung, breast and prostate, and colorectal cancer) (317,500) • Stroke (131,500)

AIDS = acquired immune deficiency syndrome; CNS = central nervous system.
*Across gender and ethnic groups

Answers to Patient Snapshot Questions

21-1. Medicare will pay this patient's hospital bill and rehabilitation facility bill (Part A) as well as the ambulance bill (Part B). Medicare will only pay for his care in the nursing home for a limited time after hospitalization. The patient himself will then use his own funds to pay for long-term nursing home care. After his own funds are used up, Medicaid will pay the costs of his care.

21-2. Of these four patients, the man from a low socioeconomic group is the one likely to be most ill when seeing a physician. Individuals in lower socioeconomic groups delay seeking treatment because of the cost; also, men are less likely to seek medical treatment than women.

22

Legal and Ethical Issues in Medical Practice

I. PROFESSIONAL BEHAVIOR

 Patient snapshot 22-1. A dermatology resident is attracted to one of his patients and would like to ask her out on a date. He only treated her once and never plans on treating her again.

Can the resident refer the patient to a colleague and then ask her out on a date? (see I B 3)

A. Impaired physicians

  1. Causes of impairment in physicians include **substance abuse,** physical or mental illness, and impairment in functioning associated with old age.

  2. Reporting of an impaired medical student (to the dean of the medical school), resident (to the residency training director) or colleague (to the state licensing board or the impaired physicians program), is **an ethical requirement** because patients must be protected and the impaired physician must be helped.

B. Medical malpractice. Physicians who are impaired may make errors in treating patients. However, physician error is not necessarily medical malpractice.

  1. The "4 D's." For a malpractice claim, the patient must prove that the physician demonstrated **dereliction,** or negligence (e.g., deviation from normal standards of care), of a **duty** (i.e., there is an established physician-patient relationship) that caused **damages** (i.e., injury) **directly** to the patient (i.e., the damages were caused by the negligence, not by another factor).
    a. Surgeons (including obstetricians) and **anesthesiologists** are the specialists most likely to be sued for malpractice. Psychiatrists and family practitioners are the least likely to be sued.
    b. Recently there has been an increase in the number of malpractice claims, due mainly to a **breakdown** of the traditional **physician-patient relationship.**

  2. Malpractice is a **tort,** or **civil wrong,** not a crime. A physician who is found guilty of malpractice may be required to pay money to compensate the patient for suffering as well as for medical bills and lost income.

  3. Romantic relationships with current or former patients are inappropriate. The patient can file an ethics complaint or a medical malpractice complaint, or both.

II. LEGAL COMPETENCE

Patient snapshot 22-2. A 22-year-old man with schizophrenia would like to enter a clinical trial for a new antipsychotic medication. The patient lives in a group home and has a part-time job.

Can the patient sign the consent form and enter the clinical trial? (see II C 2)

A. Definition

1. To be **legally competent** a patient must understand the **risks, benefits, and likely outcome** of a health care decision.

2. **All adults** (persons 18 years of age and older) are assumed to be legally competent to make their own health care decisions.

B. Minors

1. **Minors** (persons younger than 18 years of age) usually are **not** considered legally competent.

2. **Emancipated minor.** These minors are considered adults and can give consent for their own medical care. To be emancipated, they must meet any of the following criteria:
   a. They are **self-supporting** or in the **military**
   b. They are **married** or **have children** whom they care for

C. Questions of competence

1. If an adult's competence is in question (e.g., mentally retarded or demented persons), **a judge** (not the patient's family or physician) **makes the determination** of competence. Physicians are often consulted by the judge for information about whether the patient has the capacity to make health care decisions.

2. A person may meet the legal standard for competence to accept or refuse medical treatment even if she is **mentally ill or retarded** or is incompetent in other areas of her life (e.g., with finances).

III. INFORMED CONSENT

Patient snapshot 22-3. An alert 55-year-old man who is paralyzed and cannot speak requires surgery. He is informed about the procedure and, as instructed, he blinks his eyes twice for *Yes* when asked if he gives his consent.

Has the physician obtained informed consent from this patient? (see III A 1)

A. Overview

1. With the exception of life-threatening emergencies, physicians must obtain written or oral consent from competent, adult patients before proceeding with **any medical or surgical treatment.** Nonverbal responses from competent patients unable to speak or write are also acceptable.

2. Other hospital personnel (e.g., nurses) usually cannot obtain informed consent.

3. A relative (e.g., a spouse) cannot give consent to treat a patient unless the relative has a durable power of attorney or is the patient's legal guardian.

B. Components of informed consent

1. Before patients can give consent to be treated, **they must be informed of and understand the health implications** of their diagnosis. The physician can delay

telling the patient the diagnosis until she indicates that she is ready to receive the news.

2. Patients must also be informed:
   a. Of the **health risks and benefits** of treatment and the **alternatives** to treatment
   b. Of the likely **outcome if they do not consent** to the treatment
   c. That they can **withdraw consent at any time** before or during the treatment

C. Special situations

1. Competent patients have the **right to refuse to have** a needed test or procedure for religious or other reasons, even if their health will suffer or death will result from such refusal.

2. If a competent patient **requests cessation of artificial life support,** it is both legal and ethical for a physician to comply with this request.

3. Although medical or surgical intervention may be necessary to protect the health or life of the fetus, a **competent pregnant woman has the right to refuse** intervention (e.g., cesarean section, HIV testing, treatment with AZT), even if the fetus will die or be seriously injured without the intervention.

4. If an **unexpected finding** during surgery necessitates a nonemergency procedure for which the patient has not given consent (e.g., biopsy of an unsuspected ovarian malignancy during a tubal ligation), the additional procedure cannot be performed until the patient wakes up from the surgery and gives informed consent.

D. Treatment of minors

1. Only the **parent or legal guardian** can give consent for surgical or medical treatment of a minor (unless the minor is emancipated).

2. A **court order** can be obtained from a judge (within hours if necessary) if a child has a life-threatening condition or a correctable birth defect and the parent or guardian refuses to consent to an **established** (but not an experimental) medical or surgical procedure for religious or other reasons.

3. Parental consent is **not required** in the treatment of minors:
   a. In **emergency** situations when the parent or guardian cannot be located and a delay in treatment can cause harm
   b. For the treatment of **sexually transmitted diseases**
   c. For prescription of **contraceptives**
   d. For medical care during **pregnancy**
   e. For the treatment of **drug and alcohol dependence**

4. Most states require parental consent when a minor seeks an abortion.

IV. CONFIDENTIALITY

Patient snapshot 22-4. A 35-year-old man tells his physician that he has been sexually abusing his 10-year-old daughter.

Is the physician obligated to report this behavior and, if so, to whom? (see IV B)

A. In most circumstances, physicians are **expected ethically to maintain patient confidentiality.** They are not required to do so if their patient:

     1. Is suspected of child or elder abuse

     2. Has a significant risk of suicide

     3. Poses a credible threat to another person

  B. **The Tarasoff decision. According to this legal decision, if the patient poses a credible threat,** the physician must **notify** the appropriate law enforcement officials or social service agency and **warn** the intended victim.

  C. **Involuntary hospitalization**

     1. Under certain circumstances, patients with psychiatric disorders who are a **danger to themselves or others** may be hospitalized against their will (see Chapter 15).

     2. Patients who are either voluntarily or involuntarily confined to mental health facilities have the **right to receive treatment and to refuse treatment**

V. INFECTIOUS DISEASES

Patient snapshot 22-5. A physician refuses to treat a 30-year-old HIV-positive man because she is afraid of infection.

Is the physician's refusal to treat ethical? Is it legal? (see V B 2)

  A. Most states require physicians to report **varicella, hepatitis, measles, mumps, rubella, salmonellosis, shigellosis, tuberculosis, syphilis, gonorrhea, chlamydia,** and **AIDS** to their state health departments. Reporting an HIV-positive patient is required in some states.

     1. **States may differ** on which illnesses must be reported.

     2. **State health departments report** these illness (without patient names) to the federal Centers for Disease Control and Prevention (**CDC**) for statistical purposes.

  B. **HIV infection**

     1. Physicians are **not required to inform** either patients or the medical establishment about another physician's HIV-positive status; if an HIV-positive physician follows procedures for infection control, he poses no risk to his patients.

     2. Although physicians are **not compelled legally** to treat any patient, **it is unethical to refuse** to treat patients because of fear of infection, such as HIV.

     3. Patients who are HIV positive **must protect their sexual partners from infection.** If they fail to do so (i.e., if they do not use a condom or do not tell the partner of his or her HIV-positive status) and the physician has knowledge of such failure, the physician can inform the threatened partner.

VI. ADVANCE DIRECTIVES

Patient snapshot 22-6. One month after a 75-year-old woman has signed a document giving her neighbor durable power of attorney, she has a stroke. It is determined that there is little chance that she will ever regain consciousness. The patient's son, with whom she lives, insists that his mother is kept on life support. The neighbor tells the physician to remove life support.

What should the physician do? (see VI A 1)

  A. **Overview**

     1. **Advance directives** are instructions given by patients in anticipation of the need for a medical decision. A durable power of attorney and a living will are examples of advance directives.

   a. A **durable power of attorney** is a document in which a competent person **designates another person** (e.g., spouse, friend) as her legal representative to make decisions about her health care when she can no longer do so.

   b. A **living will** is a document in which a competent person gives directions for his future health care if he becomes incompetent to make decisions when he needs care.

2. Health care facilities that receive Medicare payments (i.e., most hospitals and nursing homes) **are required to ask patients** whether they have advance directives and, if necessary, **help patients** to write them.

B. Special situations

1. **The substituted judgment standard.** If an incompetent patient does not have an advance directive, health care providers or family members **(surrogates)** must determine **what the patient would have done if she were competent.** The **personal wishes of surrogates are irrelevant** to the medical decision.

2. If the patient **regains function** (competence), even briefly or intermittently, she regains the right to make decisions about her health care during those periods.

VII. DEATH AND EUTHANASIA

Patient snapshot 22-7. A terminally ill 60-year-old woman is in severe pain. The physician knows that the amount of medication required to relieve her pain will depress her respiration and potentially shorten her life.

Is it legal and ethical for the physician to administer the medication? (see VII B)

A. Legal standard of death

1. In the United States, the legal standard of death when cardiorespiratory criteria are not met, is **irreversible cessation of all functions of the entire brain,** including the brain stem.

2. If the patient is legally dead, the physician is authorized to **remove life support.** A court order or relative's permission is unnecessary.

B. **Euthanasia.** According to medical codes of ethics (e.g., American Medical Association, medical specialty organizations), **euthanasia (i.e., mercy killing, physician-assisted suicide) is a criminal act** and is never appropriate. However, it is legal and ethical to **provide medically needed analgesia** to a terminally ill patient **even if it coincidentally may shorten the patient's life.**

Answers to Patient Snapshot Questions

22-1. Romantic relationships with current or former patients are inappropriate. The resident should not ask the patient on a date now or in the future.

22-2. All adults are assumed to be legally competent to make their own health care decisions. Unless a judge has determined that this patient is incompetent, the patient himself can sign the consent form and enter the drug trial.

22-3. The physician has obtained informed consent from this patient. Nonverbal responses (e.g., eye blinks) from competent patients who are unable to speak or write are acceptable for this purpose.

22-4. Physicians are not required to maintain patient confidentiality when a patient is suspected of child abuse. The physician must report this situation to the appropriate social service agency.

22-5. This physician's refusal to treat the patient is unethical but legal. Although it is unethical to refuse to treat a patient because of fear of infection, physicians are not legally compelled to treat any patient.

22-6. The physician should follow the instructions of the neighbor. By virtue of the durable power of attorney, the patient has designated the neighbor as her legal representative to make decisions about her health care when she can no longer do so.

22-7. It is both legal and ethical for the physician to administer the medication. Although the medication may shorten the patient's life, the physician's purpose in administering it is to relieve her pain.

23

Epidemiology

I. OVERVIEW

 Patient snapshot 23-1. A town in New Jersey has a population of 7500. In the year 2001, 200 residents of the town are diagnosed with rheumatoid arthritis (RA). In the year 2002, while the town's population remains at 7500, 100 more residents are discovered to have RA.

What is the incidence rate and prevalence ratio of RA in this town in 2002? (see I B)

A. Definition. Epidemiology is the study of the factors that determine the occurrence and distribution of diseases in human populations.

B. Incidence and prevalence

   1. Incidence rate is the number of individuals who newly develop an illness in a specific time period divided by the total number of individuals at risk for the illness during that time period; for example, the number of town residents newly diagnosed with RA in 2002 divided by the total number of town residents during 2002 who are at risk for RA. That is, 100/7300. (Note: The number at risk for RA is 7500 minus the 200 residents diagnosed with RA in 2001)

   2. Prevalence ratio is the number of individuals in the population who have an illness (e.g., have RA) at a specific point in time (e.g., on March 4, 2002) or during a specific period (e.g., during 2002) divided by the total population mid-year in 2002.

   3. Relationship between incidence and prevalence
      a. Prevalence is equal to incidence multiplied by the average duration of the disease process.
      b. Prevalence is greater than incidence if the disease is long-lasting.

II. RESEARCH STUDY DESIGN

A. Research study designs include **cohort** (both prospective and historical), **case-control**, and **cross-sectional** studies (Table 23-1).

B. Clinical treatment trials

   1. These are special types of cohort studies in which some members of the group (cohort) with a specific illness are given one treatment, and other members of the cohort are given another treatment or a placebo.

   2. The results of the two treatments are then compared (e.g., differences in survival rates between men with heart disease who receive a new drug and men with heart disease who receive a standard drug are compared).

Table 23-1

Research Study Design

Type of Study	Population at the Initiation of the Study	Example
Prospective (concurrent) cohort study	Subjects who are free of illness	A study is designed to determine whether students who start to smoke at age 16 years will have more respiratory complaints by their 21st birthdays than students who do not start to smoke
Historical (nonconcurrent) cohort study	Subjects who are free of illness	A study is designed to determine whether chemical exposure 30 years ago is associated with an increased incidence of lung cancer in 2000 men who worked in a paint manufacturing plant
Case-control	Subjects who have an illness (i.e., cases) and subjects who do not have the illness (i.e., controls)	A study is designed to determine whether more women with lung cancer (cases) report a history of smoking during teenage years than women without lung cancer (controls)
Cross-sectional	Subjects studied at a specific point in time (may or may not have the illness)	A study is designed to determine whether smokers have more colds than nonsmokers according to a random telephone sample

III. RELATIVE AND ATTRIBUTABLE RISK AND THE ODDS RATIO

A. Risk factors are variables that are linked to the cause of a disease.

B. Relative risk, attributable risk, and the odds ratio are used to analyze the results of population studies (Table 23-2).

IV. TESTING. To be useful, testing instruments must be bias-free, reliable, and valid (i.e., sensitive and specific).

A. Reducing bias

1. A biased test is constructed so that one outcome is more likely than another. Placebos, blind, crossover, and randomized studies are used to reduce bias.

a. **Selection bias** can occur if subjects or investigators are permitted to choose the drug or placebo group rather than the subjects being assigned randomly.

b. **Sampling bias** can occur if factors unrelated to the aim of the study distinguish the subjects from the rest of the population (e.g., college students who volunteer for a study on cocaine use may be different from the rest of the student population).

2. **Placebo responses.** At least one third of patients respond to treatment with placebos (inert substances). In psychiatric illness, the placebo effect is even greater.

3. **Blind studies.** In a double-blind study, neither the subject nor the experimenter knows which treatment the subject is receiving.

Table 23-2
Relative Risk, Attributable Risk, and Odds Ratio

Type of Analysis	Used to analyze	Example
Relative risk	Cohort studies	If the incidence rate of lung cancer among smokers in Newark, NJ, in 1996 is 50:1000 and the incidence rate of lung cancer among nonsmokers in Newark in 1996 is 2:1000, the relative risk is 50:2, or 25. That is, the risk of lung cancer is 25 times higher for smokers than for nonsmokers.
Attributable risk	Cohort studies	Given the data above, the risk of lung cancer attributable to smoking (the attributable risk) is 50:1000–2:1000, or 48:1000. That is, 48:1000 cases of lung cancer can be attributed to smoking.
Odds ratio	Case-control studies	Of 200 patients treated in a hospital, 50 have lung cancer; of these patients, 45 are smokers; of the remaining 150 patients, 60 are smokers; the odds ratio for smoking and the risk of lung cancer is:

	Smokers	Nonsmokers
People with lung cancer	A = 45	B = 5
People without lung cancer	C = 60	D = 90

$$\frac{(A)\,(D)}{(B)\,(C)} = \frac{(45)\,(90)}{(5)\,(60)} = 13.5 = \text{Odds ratio}$$

The risk of lung cancer is 13.5 times higher for smokers than for nonsmokers in this population.

4. **Crossover studies**
   a. In a crossover study, subjects in group 1 first receive the drug and subjects in group 2 first receive the placebo.
   b. Later in the study, the groups switch (i.e., those in group 1 receive the placebo; those in group 2 receive the drug). Thus each subject acts as his or her own control.

5. **Randomization.** To ensure that the number of sick and well people is proportional in treatment and control or placebo groups, patients are randomly assigned to the groups.

B. **Reliability and validity**

1. Reliability is the reproducibility of results.
   a. **Interrater reliability** means that the results of the test are similar when the test is administered by a different rater or examiner.
   b. **Test-retest reliability** means that the results are the same when the subject is tested a second or third time.

2. **Validity** is a measure of whether the test assesses what it was designed to assess. Sensitivity and specificity are components of validity.

C. **Sensitivity and specificity** (Example 23-1)

1. **Sensitivity** measures how well a test identifies truly ill people, or true positives.

2. **Specificity** measures how well a test identifies truly well people, or true negatives.

Example 23-1. Sensitivity, Specificity, Predictive Value, and Prevalence

A new test to detect the presence of tuberculosis (TB) was given to 1000 patients. Although 200 of the patients were infected with the bacillus, the result was positive in only 160 patients (true +); the other 40 infected patients had negative results (false −) and thus were not identified by this new test. Of the 800 patients who were not infected, the result was negative in 720 patients (true −) and positive in 80 patients (false +).

Use this information to calculate the sensitivity, specificity, positive predictive value, and negative predictive value of the test and the prevalence of TB in this population.

	Patients infected with TB	Patients not infected with TB	Total patients
Positive TB test result	160 (true +)	80 (false +)	240 (those with + test result)
Negative TB test result	40 (false −)	720 (true −)	760 (those with − test result)
Total patients	200	800	1000

$$\text{Sensitivity} = \frac{160 \text{ (true +)}}{160 \text{ (true +)} + 40 \text{ (false −)}} = \frac{160}{200} = 80.0\%$$

$$\text{Specificity} = \frac{720 \text{ (true −)}}{720 \text{ (true −)} + 80 \text{ (false +)}} = \frac{720}{800} = 90.0\%$$

$$\text{Positive predictive value} = \frac{160 \text{ (true +)}}{160 \text{ (true +)} + 80 \text{ (false +)}} = \frac{160}{240} = 66.67\%$$

$$\text{Negative predictive value} = \frac{720 \text{ (true −)}}{720 \text{ (true −)} + 40 \text{ (false −)}} = \frac{720}{760} = 94.7\%$$

$$\text{Prevalence} = \frac{200 \text{ (total infected patients)}}{1000 \text{ (total patients)}} = 20.0\%$$

D. Predictive value (see Example 23-1)

    1. The **predictive value** of a test is a measure of the percentage of test results that match the actual diagnosis.

    2. **Positive predictive value** is the probability that someone with a positive test actually has the illness.

    3. **Negative predictive value** is the probability that a person with a negative test is actually well.

    4. If the **prevalence of a disease in the population is low,** even tests with very high sensitivity and specificity will have low positive predictive value.

E. Clinical probability and attack rate

    1. **Clinical probability** is the number of times an event occurs divided by the number of times that the event can occur (Example 23-2).

    2. **Attack rate** is a type of incidence rate used to describe disease outbreaks.

        a. It is calculated by dividing the number of people who become ill during the study period divided by the number of people at risk during the study period.

        b. For example, if 45 of 60 people who eat turkey and 15 of 30 people who eat steak at a banquet become ill 1 hour later, the attack rate is 75% for the turkey and 50% for the steak.

Example 23-2. Clinical Probability

After 2 years of clinical trials, it is determined that 20% of patients who take a new drug for hypertension develop nausea. If two patients (patients A and B) take the drug, calculate the following probabilities.

The probability that	Calculations
Both patients A and B will experience nausea	Multiply the probability of patient A experiencing nausea by the probability of patient B experiencing nausea: $0.20 \times 0.20 = 0.04 = 4\%$
At least one patient (i.e., either A or B *or* both A and B) will experience nausea	Add the probability of patient A experiencing nausea to the probability of B experiencing nausea and then subtract the probability of both A and B experiencing nausea (see above): $0.20 + 0.20 - 0.04 = 0.36 = 36\%$
Neither patient A nor patient B will experience nausea	Multiply the probability of patient A feeling well by the probability of patient B feeling well: $0.80 \times 0.80 = 0.64 = 64\%$

Answer to Patient Snapshot Question

23-1. The incidence of RA in 2002 is 100/7300, the number who were diagnosed with the illness divided by the number of people at risk for the illness. Because the 200 people who were diagnosed with RA in 2001 are no longer at risk for getting the illness in 2002, the denominator in this equation (the number of people at risk) is 7300 (rather than 7500). The prevalence ratio of this disease in 2002 is 300/7500. This represents the people who were diagnoses in 2002 (100 people) plus the people who were diagnosed in 2001 and still have the disease (200 people) divided by the total population.

24

Statistical Analyses

I. VARIABLES AND MEASURES OF DISPERSION AND CENTRAL TENDENCY

 Patient snapshot 24-1. Analysis of the data from a research study designed to examine the hypothesis that estrogen replacement therapy is associated with an increased risk for breast cancer reveals a p value of < 0.01.

Is this a statistically significant result? Can the researcher reject the null hypothesis? (see II B)

A. Variables

    1. A **variable** is a quantity that changes under different circumstances.

    2. Independent variables are characteristics that an experimenter can change (e.g., amount of salt in the diet).

    3. Dependent variables are outcomes that reflect the experimental change (e.g., blood pressure under different salt regimens).

B. Measures of dispersion

    1. Standard deviation (σ) is the average distance of observations from their mean. Standard deviation is obtained by squaring each variation, or deviation from the mean in a group of scores; adding the squared deviations; dividing the sum by the number of scores in the group minus 1; and determining the square root of the result.

    2. A standard normal value, or z **score,** is the difference between an individual variable and the population mean in units of standard deviation. For example:

$$z = \frac{\text{A score in the distribution} - \text{the mean score of the distribution}}{\text{The standard deviation of the distribution}}$$

    3. Standard error is the standard deviation divided by the square root of the number of scores in the set.

C. Measures of central tendency. In a group of scores:

    1. The **mean** is the average score.

    2. The **median** is the middle value when the scores are ordered sequentially.

    3. The **mode** is the value that appears most often

D. Normal distribution

    1. A **normal distribution** is also known as a **gaussian,** or **bell-shaped,** distribution. It is a theoretical distribution of scores in which the mean, median, and mode are equal (Figure 24-1).

2. In a positively or negatively **skewed distribution,** the modal peak shifts to one side (Figure 24-2).

II. HYPOTHESIS TESTING. An **hypothesis** is a statement based on inference, literature, or preliminary studies. The statement postulates that a difference exists between two groups. The possibility that the observed difference occurred by chance is tested with statistical procedures.

A. The **null hypothesis** postulates that there is no difference between the two groups. This hypothesis is either rejected or not rejected after statistical analysis.

1. **Example of the null hypothesis**
   a. A group of fifty patients who have similar serum uric acid levels at the beginning of a study (time 1) is divided into two groups of 25 patients each. One group is given daily doses of an experimental drug (experimental group). The other group is given a placebo daily (placebo group). Uric acid level is measured 4 weeks later (time 2).
   b. The null hypothesis assumes that there are no significant differences in uric acid level between the two groups at time 2.
   c. If, at time 2, patients in the experimental group show serum uric acid levels similar to those in the placebo group, the null hypothesis (i.e., there is no significant difference between the groups) is not rejected.
   d. If, at time 2, patients in the experimental group have significantly lower serum uric acid levels than those in the placebo group, the null hypothesis is rejected.

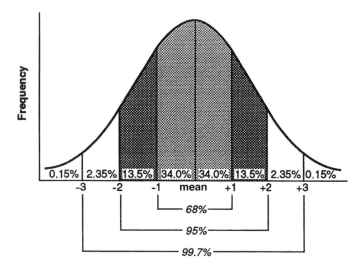

Area under the curve

Figure 24-1.   The normal (gaussian) distribution. The number of standard deviations (-3 to $+3$) from the mean is shown on the x-axis. The percentage of the population that falls under the curve within each standard deviation is shown. (From Fadem B: *BRS Behavioral Science,* 3rd ed. Baltimore, Lippincott, Williams & Wilkins, 2000, p. 255.)

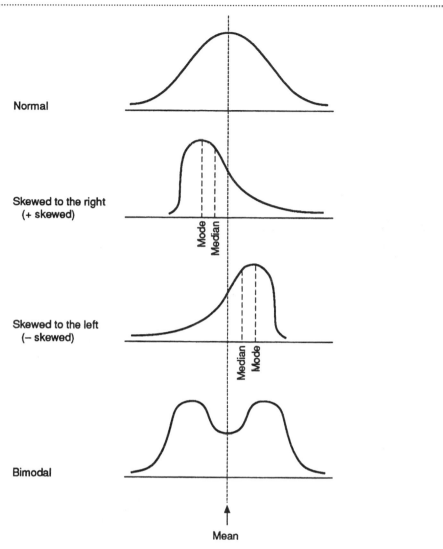

Figure 24-2. Frequency distributions. (From Fadem B: *BRS Behavioral Science*, 3rd ed. Baltimore, Lippincott, Williams & Wilkins, 2000, p. 256.)

   2. **Type I (α) and type II (β) error**
   a. α is a preset level of significance, usually set at 0.05 by convention.
   b. Power (1 minus β) is the ability to detect a difference between groups if it is truly there. The larger the sample size, the more power a researcher has to detect this difference.
   c. A **type I error** occurs when the null hypothesis is rejected even though it is true (e.g., the drug does not reduce uric acid level).
   d. A **type II error** occurs when the null hypothesis is not rejected even though it is false (e.g., the drug reduces uric acid level).
 B. **Statistical probability**
   1. The *p* (probability) value is the chance of a type I error occurring. If a *p* value is

Example 24-1. Commonly Used Statistical Tests

To evaluate the success of three commercial weight loss programs, a consumer group assigns subjects to three groups (group A, group B, and group C). The average weight of the subjects among the groups is not significantly different at the start of the study (time 1). Each group follows a different diet regimen. At time 1 and at the end of the 6-week study (time 2), the subjects are weighed and their blood pressures are obtained. Examples of how statistical tests can be used to analyze the results of this study are given below.

1. ***t*-test: difference between the means of two samples**

   Independent (nonpaired) test: Tests the difference between the mean body weights of people in group A and people in group B at time 2. Two groups of people are sampled on one occasion.

   Dependent (paired) test: Tests the difference between mean body weights of people in group A at time 1 and time 2. The same people are sampled on two occasions.

2. **Analysis of variance: differences between the means of more than two samples**

   One-way analysis: Tests the difference among mean body weights of people in group A, group B, and group C at time 2 (i.e., one variable: group).

   Two-way analysis: Tests the differences between mean body weights of men versus women and among mean body weights of group A, group B, and group C at time 2 (i.e., two variables: group and gender).

3. **Linear correlation: mutual relation between two continuous variables.** Tests the relation between blood pressure and body weight in all subjects at time 2. Correlation coefficients (*r*) are negative and range from 0 to −1 (i.e., if one variable increases as the other decreases) and are positive and range from 0 to +1 (if both variables change in the same direction).

---

equal to or less than 0.05, it is unlikely that a type I error has been made (i.e., a type I error is made five or fewer times out of 100 attempts).

2. A p value equal to or less than 0.05 (e.g., $p < 0.01$) is generally considered statistically significant.

III. STATISTICAL TESTS. Statistical tests are used to analyze data from epidemiologic studies.

   A. Parametric statistical tests are used to evaluate the presence of statistically significant differences between groups when the distribution of scores in a population is normal and when the sample size is large. Frequently used parametric statistical tests are listed in Example 24-1.

   B. Nonparametric statistical tests include Wilcoxon's (rank sum and signed-rank), Mann-Whitney, and Kruskal-Wallis tests. These tests are used when the distribution of scores in a population is not normal or the sample size is small.

   C. Categorical tests, including the **chi-square or Fisher's Exact tests,** are used to analyze categorical data or compare proportions.

Answer to Patient Snapshot Question

24-1. A p value of < 0.01 is considered to be statistically significant. The researcher can reject the null hypothesis.

Index

Note: Page numbers in *italics* indicate illustrations; those followed by t indicate tables.